'Lively and well researched . . . most of the ideas you will encounter about the menopause have been informed and distorted by the most grotesque misogyny, stretching back two and a half thousand years, which [Foxcroft] documents in forensic detail' Joan Smith, *Literary Review*

'Witty and insightful, *Hot Flushes, Cold Science* will entertain, infuriate and inspire women of all ages' *The Gloss*

'Louise Foxcroft is soooo right. There's a whole steaming pile of negative assumptions about the menopause out there . . . [this] fine and sympathetic study . . . is so much more than a book about the end of something. No: it's about how women are primarily judged by their age, and by their appearance' Rachel Johnson, *First Post*

'Foxcroft [is] good on the commercial imperatives of age and the concealment of it . . . [a] valuable contribution to an emerging literature of the third age' Claire Armitstead, *Guardian*

HOT FLUSHES, COLD SCIENCE

The History of the Modern Menopause

LOUISE FOXCROFT

GRANTA

Granta Publications, 12 Addison Avenue, London W11 4QR

First published in Great Britain by Granta Books, 2009
This paperback edition published by Granta Books, 2010

A CIP catalogue record for this book
is available from the British Library.

1 3 5 7 9 10 8 6 4 2

ISBN 978 1 84708 171 1

Printed and bound in Great Britain by CPI Bookmarque, Croydon

*For my mother, Madge,
and my boys, Tom and Jack*

CONTENTS

ACKNOWLEDGEMENTS

My heartfelt thanks to Lizzie Speller, Caron Freeborn, Fiona Green, Vic Gatrell, Suzanne Dominian, Liz Welch and Meryl Davies for all manner of things but, as far as this book goes, for their enthusiasm, encouragement, coffee, comfort and discussion. Thanks, too, to Lucy Cavendish College, Cambridge, for a brave new world; to George Miller, who first championed the idea of writing this book, and to my patient editor Bella Shand and those at Granta who have been involved. Acknowledgement is accorded to the Hosking Houses Trust for the Residency 2008 and financial support. www.hoskinghouses.co.uk. And my eternal thanks to the late Brian Outhwaite, who was much loved and is much missed.

INTRODUCTION

The 'crises' of a woman's life have been much descanted upon
by men medical writers [and] perhaps the most artificially
created has been her 'change'.

Marie Stopes, *Change of Life in Men and Women*

No one wants the menopause. It is an age under siege, riddled
with treacherous clichés and anachronisms, regularly used as
a lazy insult by the unimaginative and unthinking, and subject to an onslaught of medical treatments. Less than 300
years ago it barely existed on the medical radar, let alone
made appearances in classifications of diseases and other
works on pathology. Women had been getting on with it,
and through it, for millennia. When the menopause did
make its debut as an official medical entity in the eighteenth
century, the emphasis was on reassuring patients. But as the
menopause was illuminated, it was pathologized, and ghastly
and fatal complaints were attributed to it. For women, it
became a gateway to disappointment, disease and death.

There are many books on the shelf about 'dealing with' or
'surviving' the menopause, all presupposing you've got a fight
on your hands. Their titles, 'secret' this, 'silent' that, and
'hidden' the other, purport to oust a taboo but, in their use of

language, do more to perpetuate it. The menopause needs to be seen in its historical, medical and cultural context without polemic or self-pitying pseudo-empowerment. Very powerful medical and cultural trends have dictated women's experience of the menopause and women, in turn, have surrendered to, resisted, been complicit in or influenced these. It seems right that the menopause, being of the body, comes within the realm of medical interest, but it is a natural phenomenon and not the disease it came to be described as. Palliative treatments and management, which have a long history, are one thing, whilst interventionist, artificial attempts to circumvent, waylay or postpone the menopause are another. We must challenge prejudices instead of continuing a vain, 250-year-old attempt to pin down the menopause as a disease with the concomitant, spurious idea of a 'cure'. Attitudes to the menopause have led to therapies which are sometimes comforting, sometimes illusory and often, unfortunately, dangerous.

In Western medical orthodoxy the term 'menopause' refers specifically to the cessation of menstruation, so it can be diagnosed with any certainty only after a year's spontaneous amenorrhoea; if you haven't had a period, naturally, in the last twelve months then your last one signalled that your menopause has happened. It is understood as the most obvious manifestation of a 'gradual decline in ovarian function', a hormonal cascade which begins about five years before the last period. Described as a breakdown in the feedback mechanism of the hormonal loop between the hypothalamus, the pituitary glands and the ovaries it looks simply deterministic, riddled with regressive implications, a peculiarly female biological inevitability. But men have hormones too, and, arguably, a menopause, if we think of it as a transitional phase which is part of the ageing process.

The menopause is a phenomenon not so much hijacked by medicine as gradually occupied and authorities throughout the ages have been grimly trying, and failing, to define their subject. The Venetian physician Giovanni Marinello, writing in 1563, attributed all kinds of ills to the menopause, ills which affected almost every bodily system. If women could no longer produce babies their bodies would collapse for want of useful purpose:

> Those [women] in whom they [the periods] have stopped or do not come: like those in whom they begin to end for reasons of age, are always infirm and most of all in those parts of the body which are connected to and have some kind of correspondence with the uterus, such as the stomach and the head; thus as soon as the periods stop, pains arise, apostemata, eye disorders, weak sight, vomiting, fever . . . the disorderly uterus rises or descends all the time or commits other actions difficult to endure. From this soon a tightness of the chest arises, faintings of the heart, breathlessness, hiccups, and other troublesome accidents, from which the woman sometimes dies. Also spitting of blood, hemorrhoids, and, especially in maidens, copious nose bleeding come from it, and endless other ills, which we think too many to relate.[1]

The modern menopause has been constructed from such miserable diagnoses; it groans under centuries of cultural baggage. In classical medical opinion women were defined as deformed males who at least reverted to an approximation of the ideal of masculinity at menopause, but were said to lose their femininity, beauty, fertility, viability and their status which traditionally rested on these attributes. The beliefs of Greek and Roman physicians still formed the basis of Western medical thought in the eighteenth century, infusing the beginnings of medical science and the first works written specifically on the menopause. Modern attitudes to the menopause arise directly out of a poisonous history of lack and loss, disease and decay.

Though attitudes and treatments have changed over time, the menopause remains an inevitable constant. It's not a question of choice. This significant but very ordinary life event will affect half the population. Already one third of the female population in Western societies is experiencing it.[2] Globally, there will be up to 1.2 billion post-menopausal women after 2030, about 10 per cent of the world's population, and a further 25 million will reach the menopause each year thereafter.[3] Yet why do we think of the menopause in the way we do – often with dread and distaste? Its rich historical, social and cultural context is to blame: it has been mediated through medicine from antiquity to the present, and current attitudes and treatments have been reached through the filter of thousands of years of rampant chauvinism, collusion, trial, error and secrecy. Women's actual and fictional experiences, describing their perspective on the menopause through time, are less easy to come by. The views, experiences, resistances or otherwise to the menopause and its medical interpretation reveal the informative, speculative, philosophical and emotional responses of anger, curiosity, shame, fear and sometimes indifference, relief and pleasure. And the language used to describe the menopause is far from an innocent representation of the condition – its shades of meaning construct as well as reflect understanding.[4]

This is a particularly resonant moment to be exploring attitudes to the menopause. New research is emerging all the time about the benefits or otherwise of hormone replacement therapy (HRT);[5] the media reports frequently cases of women defying nature, having assisted conceptions in their fifties and even sixties (where once the doctors gave them only orgasms now they give them life using younger women's pre-menopausal eggs);[6] the recent emergence of the grandmother hypothesis — an explanation for menopause based on the older non-breeding woman helping the next generation to survive — and the advent of menopausal baby boomers, who believed they would be potent and lubricious for ever and are now the new role models for the ageing process. Even in our feminist era, if you think you are not defined by your reproductive potential, if you think that sounds too baldly biological and that of course you are more than your sex, then look at society's emphasis on youth and beauty and how it despises signs of age. Witness the horror and furore when a woman in her fifties or older behaves in a sexual way and lets on that she still likes sex and wants it.[7] Whereas a man's old age has been traditionally understood as a social process which begins with retirement, a woman's has been firmly tied to a biological process, her menopause.[8]

Ageing is undeniably biological but our negative perceptions of the processes that accompany it need addressing. Historically, it might have showed in a moustache, revealed in the 'manliness' of the three witches in *Macbeth*: 'you should be women, and yet your beards forbid me to interpret that you are so'. Or in a toothless mouth: Lady Sarah Cowper had 'but three teeth besides stumps' by the time she was seventy-one in 1715. Or in the skin, in a stoop, or in broken bones due to calcium loss: older women were 'lame, ympotente' and often carried the 'dowager's hump' of osteoporosis. 'Such is the feebleness,' wrote Lady Sarah

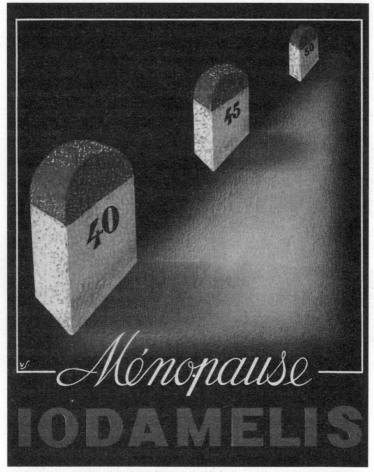

An advertisment for Iodamelis, a mid-nineteenth-century proprietary menopausal medication, looking like nothing so much as a series of tombstones stretching into a dark and forbidding future.

Cowper, 'made contemptible by crump shoulders, hips and back.' Yet we are aged by culture, by class, race, gender and access to resources.[9] It is partly the cult of youth, amongst other economic and material forces, that drives ageism. Gerontologists have been exploring the way people's bodily age might differ from how old they actually feel and have found, unsurprisingly, that one can feel older or younger than one's chronological age depending on health, well-being, environment, status and more. In fact, they suggest that bodily age and 'feel age' rarely match, and it is often hard to identify with a chronological age. How chronological age relates to a specific ageing process such as the menopause will influence how women, and men, regard and experience this transition, how their doctors will make decisions in their treatments, and how it might dictate medical research. Some women might prefer the menopause to disappear but many women might want to keep it as a significant marker in life, like a badge earned, a status achieved or a reason for a turning point in the course of their lives. In *Old Age* (1970) Simone de Beauvoir said that there is only one solution if growing older is not to be an 'absurd parody of our former life and that is to go on pursuing ends that give our existence meaning – devotion to individuals, to groups or to causes, social, political, intellectual, or creative work'.

Compare that with the story Cicely Hamilton told in *Marriage as a Trade* (1912) in which a young girl is given the benefit of an older man's opinion that all women over fifty should be shot. The effect was to

rouse in her a sense of insult . . . that she and her like should only be supposed to exist so long as they were pleasing . . . I know others who have felt the same rush of anger . . . as they recognized that character, worth, intellect were held valueless in women, that nothing counted in her but the one capacity.

And still, in the mid twentieth century, the American physician David Reuben could argue in his bestseller *Everything You Always Wanted to Know About Sex* (1969) that, 'as estrogen is shut off, a woman becomes as close as she can to being a man . . . having outlived their ovaries, they have outlived their usefulness as human beings'.

Age, beauty and worth are central themes in writings on the menopause, and feminists (de Beauvoir, Wolf, Greer, Orbach, et al.) have rightly and richly delved into them. In her 1978 essay 'The double standard of ageing' Susan Sontag wrote, 'All women are trained to want to continue looking like girls,' and 'Women grow old but men mature.'[10] Susie Orbach, in her recently updated introduction to *Fat is a Feminist Issue* (2006), has said that 'body hatred is becoming a major export of the western world' with female identity now hopelessly inextricable from body image, something that is evident every time one opens a magazine or switches on the television. Prejudice against and denigration of the older woman have been rife.

Categorizing menopausal women is a meaningless endeavour when you think of those who cross the boundaries: the menopausal yet sexual mothers of young children; those who might not be grandmothers until their seventies or even eighties; women who undergo an artificial early menopause as part of cancer treatment; women, heterosexual or lesbian, who didn't have or didn't want children; women who are very glad that they don't have to deal with periods any longer or worry about being pregnant; those who have had enough of the sexual merry-go-round or who want to get back on it; women who can now just damn well be themselves and please themselves.

A friend of mine, standing in a supermarket check-out queue idly reading the magazine headlines whilst waiting the endless wait, noted this one: *What You MUST Know About The Menopause Now.* The absurd urgency struck her, 'Now, as in before your uterus drops out in the queue, no doubt,' she thought, rumly. She noticed that the magazine offered assistance on how to get through the menopause, in case you might somehow get hopelessly stuck in it. Women must refuse to get stuck, or be regarded as stuck, or be interpreted by others according to some outmoded cultural dictates. In *Revolution from Within* Gloria Steinem wrote about the 'importance of moving closer to the true self, regardless of our age', and 'an understanding that to fear aging is to fear a new stage of life'.[11] She had heard 'fifty' as old when applied to other people and had consciously and constantly had to revise her own assumptions. For Steinem the menopause turned out to be 'mainly the loss of a familiar marker of time, plus the discomfort of a few flushes and flashes', and what it brought was a 'much-longed-for era of relative peace and self-expression'. You can age successfully, as Betty Friedan says in her book *The Fountain of Age* (1993), without conforming to the Western ideal of the serenely stolid, spiritual, asexual older woman who cares not a fig for the hurly-burly of the *chaise-longue*.

When I started thinking about the menopause, I experienced a slight but definite feeling of self-consciousness and realized that I, too, had negative assumptions about it. It is not a straightforward experience to face people's discomfort when the menopause is mentioned. When describing this book to others, I initially felt a mixture of defiance and defensiveness; I was embarrassed by the subject and would blush, then feel intensely irritated. There was usually a politely suppressed spasm of alarm, a fleeting look of distaste, and often genuine surprise, if not shock, at the very thought. Responses varied depending on age and gender: when I told my octogenarian father I was working on a history of the menopause his reaction was awkward and slightly cross; in comparison my 28-year-old son was full of questions and showed not a shred of embarrassment. It's possible that he might start a family in his thirties or later with a partner of a similar age and they'll need to be aware of fertility, so his interest seems sensible if not immediately obvious. From women in their forties and over, with one or two notable exceptions, there was a string of eager questions and strongly held opinions.

The menopause was obviously nothing to do with me when, at forty-two, I saw a doctor for some symptom he couldn't fathom. He suggested that I might be perimenopausal, the stage which precedes menopause. I was taken aback, appalled at the idea. How dare he suggest I was heading over the hill of fecundity and so, as I imperfectly understood it, desirability? I was dependent on his opinion despite my suspicion of his bluff ignorance. He was wrong anyway, had made a painful stab in the dark, but had raised all manner of conflicting thoughts, feelings and questions within me, not least on mortality.

A teenager in the 1970s, liberated and travelled, a mother at twenty-one by the end of the decade, a feminist who defiantly breastfed her babies in public, I had been fearless about sex and bodies, about my pregnancies, my 'peculiar female illnesses', yet now I found I had to wrestle with an element of antipathy within myself. The menopause seemed, unlike anything I had encountered before, a much more private, even shameful, thing to go through. Its negative image had seeped into my mind and I deeply resent that.

I can't ask my mother about the menopause as she died when I was thirty-six, long before I had begun to think about it. I vaguely remember her having her menopause in her mid-fifties, but she didn't speak about it, either because it was an easy time or because of some shame or embarrassment. I certainly hope it wasn't the latter. Maybe she discussed it with her friends or sister. Perhaps her silence was due to a private grief at losing her fertility; an unwelcome sign of ageing and a perceived loss of sexual validity. Perhaps she saw her future mapped out, shanghaied by her own body, experiencing feelings similar to those some of us have during pregnancy, of being taken over, subject to alien invasion, of not being in control of our bodies. Women feel many things when they begin their periods or become pregnant, including pleasure, anxiety, shame and pride, but few are openly proud of having the menopause.

When the menopause happens to me, I wonder if life will change drastically. Will my place in the world alter when I am no longer a fertile woman? Will I feel bereft at the loss, as if happiness is contingent upon fecundity? Or maybe the loss will be cathartic and beget freedom, excitement and relief. Perhaps desirability won't be important any longer – quite a leap to make given our cultural and biological drive to that end. Will I be waving a physical flag at everyone, like when I was heavily pregnant – an unavoidable sign of something most private made public? Pregnancy, bleeding, hot flushes – all are outward signs of the female self, signs of our sex, and they force societies, not to mention individuals, to deal with the extraordinary questions of human sexuality which, let's face it, many people still do not want to confront.

In one of the many conversations I have had about the menopause recently, a friend of mine told me that she had been out at lunch with five women, all in their early- to mid-fifties, all handsome, interesting women; one doctor, one teacher, two writers, one therapist. One had stitches from having her eyes done, one had a jaw lift planned, all had had Botox occasionally. All found their sex drive less driven, yet all owned vibrators, all were thinking and discussing with vigour how to get older when they had no models – things had changed so much from our mothers' generation, medically, cosmetically, culturally and socioeconomically. How women feel about all this and how much they surrender or resist the concomitants of ageing – whatever they perceive those to be – is the future of the menopause. There is such a great desire to know what the menopause is, what it is like, what it does, and especially what it means to the peri-menopausal, the menopausal and the post-menopausal. This history redresses the myths a woman gleans of menopause in her twenties, thirties, forties and fifties and attempts to capture the truths about this liminal state.

A post-menopausal woman asked me if I had had my menopause and said to me, 'You wait!' And I will, but I hope without the trepidation, dread or disgust that the physician John Fothergill identified and perhaps perpetuated over 200 years ago when he wrote, 'There is a period in the life of females to which, for the most part, they are taught to look with some degree of anxiety.'[12]

1

THE MODERN MENOPAUSE

Have you any notion of how many books are written about women . . . have you any notion how many are written by men . . . are you aware that you are, perhaps, the most discussed animal in the universe?

Virginia Woolf, *A Room of One's Own* (London, 1929)

The female body in medicine has been defined almost exclusively by male doctors. Overwhelmingly their attitudes have been mired in contradiction, negativity, undisguised disgust and worse. Menopausal and post-menopausal women 'desire the male more than ever', wrote the physician Giovanni Marinello in 1563, yet almost exactly four hundred years later Dr Robert Wilson, author of the bestselling *Feminine Forever*, declared that they were all 'castrates'.[1] The difference between these two statements reveals the continually changing perceptions, judgements and knowledge of what the menopause is; they do not clarify, instead they show the confusion, assumption and wild speculation that have always accompanied the phenomenon. And this is if we even accept that a syndrome called 'menopause' actually exists, rather than just the fact of the cessation of menses. No wonder the middle-aged woman feels beleaguered. The message doesn't change: it is her lot to suffer.

Although the Greeks and Romans wrote about the menopause it was viewed as a state of lack, and it is difficult to find as a medical entity – which is how we view the menopause today – before the eighteenth century. The literature is sparse, but the subject was fast becoming of interest to physicians by the time John Fothergill published his marvellous and generous study, *'Of the management proper at the cessation of the menses'*, in 1774. He was attempting to answer some of the discomforts and complaints of his older female patients (though most women went through it without the intervention of a costly physician) and to educate younger, inexperienced male doctors. At this stage the menopause was still deemed and treated as a natural phenomenon, one which might or might not need management depending on the individual crasis, the 'temperament', of the woman. It wasn't at that point thought of as a disease, and although Fothergill framed it less than positively, his emphasis was on reassurance.

Over the following 200 years, the menopause came to be seen by physicians as the gateway to disease and death. It is hardly surprising, given this history, that if women know nothing else about it, they have been taught to fear the menopause. First and foremost we have imbibed a sense of anxiety about it. The earliest medical works on the menopause take this anxiety for granted; an assumption which continues today: a young, male historian stated in 1999 that 'most women' in Western societies 'dread the effects' of the menopause, so perpetuating this perverse myth and maintaining a lucrative fear.[2] Fear of the menopause is something we have learned, and it has grown out of a general, male and medical distaste for the idea of the menopause perceived as an end of viability, fertility, beauty, desirability and worth. Since the French physician de Gardanne coined the new term '*ménèspausie*' in the early nineteenth century, an onslaught of opinion, aetiology, treatments and, not least and lest we forget, profit has followed. Women need to unlearn their dread and recognize that the menopause is not, of itself, dread-full; that we are not merely the victims of our biological selves.

The Western clinical model puts the average age at menopause at fifty-one years but it most often happens between the ages of forty-five and fifty-five – known as the climacteric era. If it happens before a woman turns forty it is defined as a premature menopause. The peri-menopause describes the time from when, as orthodox medicine describes it, 'the ovaries start to fail'; from when a woman experiences irregular periods, or hot flushes begin, until the twelve months after her final period. Menopausal transition describes the time from when the peri-menopause begins until the final period. Bleeding can gradually fade out or can become prolonged and heavy before suddenly stopping altogether. This whole process might last up to four years and starts, on average, at 47.5 years. Some 10 per cent of women cease menstruation abruptly and don't go through a long transition at all, whilst some may experience it over a period of many years. If a woman has not had a period for the two years before she reaches fifty or for one year after that birthday, then she is considered free of the likelihood of pregnancy. The post-menopause is defined as the time that follows the permanent cessation of menstruation, after a year has passed with no period, but it can be obscured if the woman is taking

HRT during her peri-menopause. It is generally estimated that about 80 per cent of women are post-menopausal by the age of fifty-four and that the same number will have experienced some symptoms. This terminology covers a broad spectrum of experience, much of which is interpreted by women through a multitude of subjective responses: physical, psychological and cultural. The menopause varies from woman to woman, race to race, culture to culture.

Some argue that the trigger for the menopause is when the ovaries begin to run out of eggs and that 'reproductive ageing' is subject to their decreasing quality and quantity. Though this is a highly plausible argument supported by clinical and experimental observations, it is still impossible to prove conclusively without removing the entire ovary.[3] A follicle, the small membranous pouch that will contain a developing oocyte, or egg, begins its development when the baby girl is only four months in the womb; by the fifth month she has a maximum of about 7 million eggs. This pool of immature follicles then begins to decline so that by the time she is born each of the child's ovaries contains from 266,000 to 472,000 follicles, and each of these contains an unformed oocyte. The decline in their numbers continues throughout her childhood so that, by the time she begins her periods, she may have about 500,000 left. Depletion carries on at a rate of about 1000 a month during her reproductive life due to atresia, a process of reabsorption, or through pregnancy. After she has reached the age of around thirty-five the rate of loss increases until the menopause. From puberty to the menopause the eggs may reach full maturity and the woman ovulates, but only about 400 follicles will ever get this far.[4]

Another theory emphasizes hypothalamic ageing as the cause of the menopause: a breakdown in the secretion of hormones by the hypothalamus leading to menopause-related events and experiences. However, medical science is still largely in the dark about the endocrine mechanisms – the system of secreting glands within the body – which dictate the cascade of hormones throughout a woman's life. The endocrine function is closely regulated by the hypothalamic feedback system, a loop of activity which encompasses the hypothalamus and pituitary glands in the brain, and the ovaries. The hypothalamus is involved in the control of endocrine function, the autonomic nervous system, body temperature, sleep, appetite, water balance, emotion and sexuality. The hypothalamus was discovered by Joseph Lieutaud in 1742, though the investigation of the circulation between it and the pituitary gland began only 200 years later, in the 1930s. This gland, the most complex of the endocrine glands, is attached by a stalk to the hypothalamus. It was once believed to drain phlegm from the brain, which gave it its name: 'pituita', meaning slime, mucus. This was refuted in the seventeenth century and, though the gland was accurately described in 1838, its function was unknown until the early twentieth century.[5] The anterior lobe of the pituitary, regulated by the hypothalamus, secretes a number of important hormones, including follicle stimulating hormone (FSH) and luteinising hormone (LH) which cause ovulation. LH is also involved in the subsequent formation of the corpus luteum, so named by the Italian physician Marcello Malpighi in 1697 because of its yellow appearance in the cow. It is a mass of progesterone-secreting endocrine tissue that forms immediately after ovulation from the ruptured follicle and it prepares the endometrium, the lining of the womb, for the implantation of the fertilized ovum. If there is a pregnancy the corpus luteum gets bigger and secretes progesterone; if not, it will atrophy and the prepared endometrium is shed in menstruation. Only a mature follicle secretes enough oestrogen to stimulate the hypothalamo-pituitary mechanism into discharging sufficient LH so the follicle will rupture and corpora lutea will form. And the mechanism by which a follicle is selected for ovulation remains one of the most mysterious of biological occurrences.

FSH and LH are secreted in response to stimulation by the gonadotrophin-releasing hormone (GnRH) from the hypothalamus, which is released in pulses so that the ovary is exposed to a fluctuating rather than a constant concentration of hormones.[6] The ovary itself, the 'biological clock', determines the length of the menstrual cycle, and its production of hormones ensures that there are healthy eggs ready for fertilization. In a mature woman each ovary weighs about 8 grams, but its relative size changes throughout the cycle because it is made up of transitory structures such as the follicles and corpora lutea. The post-menopausal ovary is much smaller than that which is still engaged in reproductive life because it has no functioning follicles or corpora lutea.[7] At birth LH and FSH secretions in a female are almost the same as they are when she reaches puberty, but a year or so later this calms down, and the levels are undetectable until puberty and the reactivation of GnRH. When the menopause is reached there is a final change and the levels of FSH and LH become extremely high, increasing over fifty-fold, because of the changes in the hormone feedback mechanism in the hypothalamic circuit.[8] Whichever theory or mechanism is applied, the menopausal transition is not an abrupt change: there is an acceleration in the rate of follicle loss, mainly genetically determined, in the ten years or so prior to menopause.[9]

The menopause made its debut as a medical entity in the early nineteenth century, and as it was illuminated it was pathologized. It was brought firmly within the parameters of diseases peculiar to women, and the idea that it could precipitate any number of ghastly and sometimes fatal complaints was constantly reiterated. The all-inclusive lists of physical and psychological symptoms associated with menopause today may or may not include hot flushes, cold sweats, night sweats, weight gain, backache, tingling, fatigue, headache, palpitations, arthralgia, dizzy spells, irritability, nervousness, anxiety, apathy, depression, early wakening, emotional instability, fears, feelings of suffocation, forgetfulness, insomnia, lack of concentration, lightheadedness, loss of interest, loss of self-worth, feelings of panic, sadness, tenseness, osteoporosis, depression, dysuria, dyspareunia, parasthesia, chest pains, breast pains, constipation, diarrhoea, facial hair, vaginal dryness, changes in libido, in skin and hair, and, unsurprisingly in light of these lists, worry about the body.[10] These myriad symptoms take in every bodily system – vasomotor, cardiovascular, metabolic, sensory, digestive, skeletal, glandular and the central nervous system – yet the only universally agreed symptom is vasomotor, the constriction of blood vessels which precipitates hot flushes.

This long and exhaustive list has been elaborated on since physicians first began to concentrate on the menopause in the eighteenth century, firmly establishing the idea that the phenomenon is more concerned with pathology than with healthy 'normality'. The use of the word 'symptom' implies a medical condition if not an illness or disease. Yet the definition of a symptom is mutable. Is it necessarily something to get worried about? Biomedical models tend to see changes in women's physiology as negative and in need of 'curing'.

Women themselves may note the changes in their bodies but may see them as just one more experience or even as a positive one. The word 'symptoms' can be misleading and it is questionable whether there are any menopausal symptoms besides hot flushes. As the menopause coincides with other experiences of ageing it is all the more difficult to interpret and distinguish because no one can say which symptoms are strictly menopausal and which symptoms simply parallel the process.[11] Each of the possible experiences and sensations on the endless list is associated with peri-menopause, menopause and post-menopause and placed in an unruly cascade of events from birth to death. The definitions are even now constantly being argued about and the accumulated knowledge is still incomplete because all these symptoms can have any number of other causes.

There is a persuasive argument that vasomotor disturbances, the hot flushes and night sweats linked to changes in the hypothalamic loop, are the only true features of the menopause, and these are idiosyncratic.[12] During a hot flush the blood vessels dilate, increasing the flow of blood to the skin, most noticeably to the face, neck and chest. A rise in temperature is accompanied by sensations of sometimes overwhelming heat, sweating and then cooling down, with the possibility of feeling dizzy, faint and sick. Even though hot flushes are almost synonymous with the menopause these disturbances are not experienced by all women: up to nearly 40 per cent do not have them at all. Of those who do, about 70 per cent experience them for a year, 30 per cent for about five years, and 5–10 per cent for ten years. These figures relate to European and North American women and studies in other cultures reveal marked differences: an Australian study found that only up to 25 per cent of women experience vasomotor disturbances. Hot flushes also vary enormously in intensity and length in different women, lasting for just two or three minutes or for up to an hour, and they might happen very occasionally or several times in a day.[13] Night sweats, if you get them, also vary in intensity and length. At their worst, you may have to change the sheets. After an oophorectomy, the surgical removal of the ovaries which causes an induced menopause, most women will experience hot flushes straight away whatever age they are. About 90,000 hysterectomies are carried out in Britain each year and oophorectomy takes place in about 14 per cent of these, mainly in women aged over fifty and even though their ovaries may be healthy. The usual reason given is that ovarian cancer is difficult to diagnose and that surgery may prevent future disease. It is hard to imagine a man having his testicles chopped off to avoid an illness at a later date which may or may not happen anyway. Research suggests that approximately 50 per cent of ovaries cease to function after hysterectomy.[14]

If they have hot flushes, many women can ignore them as minor inconveniences; some find them more difficult because they are a physical sign of the menopause and open one up to negative cultural interpretations. Flushing is similar to blushing with its connotations of shame, embarrassment and the desire to run. It has been suggested that the randomly occurring hot flush can trigger at the very least a symbolic lack of control which might heighten a sense of vulnerability in some women, and this perceived 'weakness' could be exacerbated by other menopausal characteristics.[15]

Osteoporosis, a gradual thinning of the bones, has become another well-entrenched fear for many mid-life women. The anxiety is that, even if it is not inevitable, it is a highly likely

misery of getting older. Yet osteoporosis is not a problem
specific to menopause, despite its strong link with the promotion of HRT. Taking the drugs to prevent bone loss is
successful only if HRT is used long term, which in itself carries many inherent risks. The prevalent idea is that women
suffer a dramatic loss of hormones at the menopause, damaging bones, but both men and women experience a gradual
decrease in levels of respective sex hormones as they age, and
they continue to produce small amounts throughout their
lives. Osteoporosis is not a gender-specific disease, as all
women and men have some risk of developing it as they grow
older. It is one consequence of ageing, and some people are
more susceptible than others. As noted by J. Gold in 1986,

> Nature did not make a mistake in ceasing ovarian estrogen
> production after the reproductive years, or by giving women
> smaller bones, or by limiting calcium absorption with age, or
> even by allowing bones to thin. On the contrary, osteoporo-
> sis is simply a long-term negative side-effect of a very positive
> survival strategy; a strategy that draws calcium from the
> bones to the blood so that the body can live. Nature provided
> us with the capacity for accumulating tremendous bone
> mineral reserve, so that we would always have both lifelong
> strong bones and a constant source of minerals for transfer to
> the blood in times of need. We, however, have outdone our-
> selves in accumulating ways to deplete our bones of their
> precious stores of life-supporting minerals.[16]

Bone consists of collagen fibres which are tough and elastic,
and minerals, predominantly calcium phosphate, which are
hard and gritty. It is constantly removed and new bone is
constantly formed; maximal bone density is reached at about

thirty years of age, and thereafter bone loss gradually exceeds bone formation. This gradual thinning of the bones is variable but where there is a severe loss of bone mineral density, most commonly affecting the hip, wrist or vertebrae, bones may break much more easily than normal, perhaps just from the impact of a fall to the ground.[17] It is estimated that up to one in three women and one in twelve men over fifty will fracture a bone due to osteoporosis, and that women develop bone loss about three times as quickly as do men.[18] About 80 per cent of our 'bone health' is inherited, which means that the other 20 per cent can be influenced through diet and exercise. The condition is slow to develop and symptoms, when they appear, include loss of height, persistent back pain, and a bent and stooping posture – one of the archetypal physical attributes of the old witch.

The National Osteoporosis Society says that most available drug treatments are only licensed to treat post-menopausal women because osteoporosis affects them more than any other group, and the pharmaceutical companies will always want to trial new drugs on this group assuming that members of it will be their biggest consumers. HRT is no longer the first treatment for osteoporosis; instead the most common drugs are bisphosphonates, which act on bone-making cells to restore some lost bone, help to prevent further bone loss and reduce the risk of fractures. Osteoporosis is less common in men because they tend to build stronger bones, though in nearly half of all men with osteoporosis the cause is unknown. But if their osteoporosis is found to be caused by low levels of testosterone, known as hypogonadism, doctors may prescribe this hormone for them.[19]

Diet is known to play a large part in the development of osteoporosis, so if serious dieting has been a constant in a woman's life, or if she has or has had anorexia nervosa or bulimia, which often means that oestrogen levels have been low for long periods of time, then she is at greater risk.[20] Excessive exercise will also exacerbate the condition, though moderate weight-bearing activities such as walking and dancing can help by strengthening the muscles around the bones. Factors which are said to increase the risk include a strong family history of osteoporosis, indicating a genetic predisposition; infrequent menstrual periods; prolonged use of steroid drugs and certain medical conditions (such as an over-active thyroid or any condition that leads to a sedentary life); smoking; drinking; a poor diet lacking in calcium or vitamin D.[21] Bone density loss is just another consequence of ageing and being post-menopausal is just one of the factors that increases a person's risk of osteoporosis. It does not mean that a woman is gradually and inevitably going to turn into the crook-backed crone of folklore, though she is a figure who is proving surprisingly hard to shake off.

This withered, ghastly and undesirable creature can be glimpsed behind many a modern account of what menopause means to women, especially where sex is concerned. Elizabeth Abbott, author of *A History of Celibacy* (2001), argues that in North America 'many aging [women] retire from sexual service', and they do this, she confidently states, 'without the slightest regret'. It is hard to read these suggestions without being struck by the use of words such as 'retire' and 'service', as if sex has been some sort of below-stairs job involving some pretty grubby chores and now it is time to hang up your boots and duster and fade silently away. Some of these women, she goes on, 'consider sex as purely for reproduction, while some say that, at their age, it is no longer necessary, proper, or dignified'. Many say they stop having sex because of illness, though the 'medical reality is that their arthritis, heart disease, or hypertension does not require it. In fact, their newly adopted celibacy may disguise or excuse antipathy to sex'.[22] There is certainly little human feeling amongst the 'mechanics' and the 'service', and no mention of the menopause or the fact that some women experience a surge in their sexual response at this time. Changes in sexual response, one way or the other, may happen gradually or suddenly but can also be attributed to ageing or the effects of being in a long-term relationship. Current works on the menopause seem to display either a dismissive attitude to historical knowledge about the subject or they just omit it altogether as irrelevant to new research.

A cursory glance at the history of female sexuality reveals the roots of our cultural taboos. We are prey to the destructive nature of the myths and prejudices we have inherited and now, more than ever before, to any potentially harmful and commercially driven interest.[23] The most intransigent myths have it that where women experience sexual 'dysfunction' it is usually a psychogenic problem and that older women have little, diminishing or no interest in sex.[24] This idea can be traced back to the nineteenth century, and even Alfred Kinsey, biologist and author of influential books on human sexuality in the late 1940s and early 1950s, thought that 'female instance of coitus was dependent on the male's sexual behavior'.[25] Such opinions have become self-fulfilling and harmful prophecies, and carry all the accompanying fears and anxieties that these perpetrate and foster in individuals. The idea, suggested by gynaecology or menopause clinical studies, that the menopause has a particularly detrimental effect on women's sexual health or enjoyment, is not supported by general population surveys.[26]

Women's sexuality is highly contextual, subject to relationships, environment, health, past experience – perhaps almost too many influences to list – yet definitions of any female sexual disorders are based mainly and narrowly on 'genitally focused events in a linear sequence model', i.e. desire, arousal and orgasm.[27] It is obvious to any woman that these definitions are totally inadequate and need revising so that they reflect women's reasons and incentives for having sex, reasons which go beyond the first feelings of desire and arousal. How can it be possible to define dysfunction and make clear distinctions between 'normal' and 'abnormal' responses, or effectively integrate the personal and subjective with objective information? The subtleties of sexual response, the slightest moves, sounds or sensations that arouse a woman or turn her off, cannot be scientifically measured or evaluated and any attempt to do so would be clumsy and distort the reality. The undeniable sexualization of society has undoubtedly muddied people's expectations and understanding of sexuality, homogenized it into a looks- and performance-oriented, one-trick-pony parody, when it is a much deeper and rarer creature.

The vagaries and differences experienced in arousal should not necessarily lead to a diagnosis of sexual dysfunction, yet many menopausal women find themselves caught in this clinical trap. The mind, a powerful and often overwhelming force in arousal, is absent from diagnoses based on 'reduced lubrication capability', 'narrowing of the vaginal vault', 'reduced androgen levels, aging of multiple body systems, and side-effects of medication'. A more arid take on arousal would be hard to find. Treatment, a given if a woman is not functioning according to cultural dictates of sexuality, has progressed only so far as a recommendation that it be based on a 'comprehensive evaluation and consideration of medical and psychosocial contributors to the individual's dysfunction'.[28]

Any debate on dysfunction falls back on arbitrary notions and the common acknowledgement that it is difficult to understand what libido really is – the *OED* suggests 'a psychic drive or energy, particularly that associated with the sexual instinct, but also that inherent in other instinctive mental desires and drives'. The physiological basis of the libido is hazy, to say the least. Some prominent clinicians continue to argue that its loss or diminution 'is a common, distressing but treatable condition in the menopausal woman' and recommend 'oestrogen with or without testosterone [as] the first-line treatment'.[29] However, oestrogen, testosterone, progesterone and various other hormones may not influence women's sexual function at all – their actions are so complex and our knowledge so incomplete. The freely available NHS Clinical Knowledge Summaries state that 'HRT has no proven direct effect on sexuality or libido', but also maintain that 'loss of libido can be improved by testosterone supplementation, particularly after surgical menopause'. Advising that women seek out specialist advice because of 'a wide range of doses, with potentially serious adverse effects', they suggest that 'the partial androgenic effects of tibolone may be useful for some women . . . an alternative to HRT for relieving vaginal dryness, significantly increasing sexual fantasies, arousability and coital frequency'.[30] Despite all the research the results are severely compromised because of the lack of agreed and validated measures of sexual function.[31]

What if a woman is quite content with a lowering of her libido? Undoubtedly, this is how sexuality can sometimes be when you are older, no longer 'fully available', not centred on the lives and needs of others, and able to experience a more reflective sexual response. Physiological and psychological changes which occur around the time of menopause may arise from other life events involving partners, work, children, elderly parents, status, quality of sleep and health. Attempts to maintain levels of 'aggressive sexual desire' through drugs may be incompatible with other aspects of mid-life experience. Individual responses are, at the very least, marginalized by science.

There is rapid growth in numbers of women coming up to the menopause and who will spend a larger proportion of their lives as post-menopausal, yet the nature, incidence and prevalence of changes in their sexual lives and function in the course of the menopausal transition and after it are poorly understood.[32] It is enormously difficult to design and carry out studies that can measure experience over time and can distinguish changes due to the menopause from changes due to general ageing. Because reproductive life is connected to sexual life the two are easily and too often conflated. Older women often retain their desire for sex and their responses can be heightened by not having to worry any longer about pregnancy and childbirth. Freedom is a well-documented aphrodisiac.

Much of the research on menopause and sex reiterates the negative assumptions about the physical, emotional and sexual changes that *may* happen, such as vaginal dryness and decreased libido. It concentrates mainly on heterosexual women and neglects the role of culture in women's responses. Women's sexual activity has traditionally been understood and measured by the frequency of penetrative intercourse and sexual satisfaction, and it assumes a pretty one-dimensional definition, constructed by a male-dominated culture.

Heterosexuality in this context implies a lot more than male–female desire, it is also an institution that helps to define society, and heterosexual menopausal women tend to describe their sex lives in ways that are bound up with this cultural mindset. But where is the research about the positive and beneficial changes that women can and do experience, the increased sexual activity, desire and orgasm intensity? A recent study in America that addressed this anomaly asked not how or whether women experienced menopausal changes, but how they *viewed* any changes in their sex lives. It gave a quite different perspective on the question. Entrenched cultural expectations about the menopause, gender and heterosexuality influence women's experience of biological changes, and moving the goalposts subtly changes the categorizations of what is normal and what is dysfunctional.[33]

Research conducted with menopausal lesbians shows that this group, who are used to thinking about themselves and their lives outside of mainstream culture, are less constrained by cultural expectations than heterosexual women. The type of sex they have affects their experiences of, for example, vaginal dryness; a male partner's assumptions about the menopause and decline may differ from a female partner's. If a woman has vaginal dryness and expects, or is expected, to have intercourse rather than another sort of sex, she will probably experience discomfort and express less interest. She might then talk about her discomfort in terms of a poor and uncommunicative relationship rather than of menopausal change. Most women in the study emphasized cultural and social issues, such as relationship status and quality, communication, willingness to change, health, sexual history and definitions of sex, rather than the menopause when they described their post-menopausal sex lives. They discuss sex in the panorama of their lives rather than in the context of any specific physiological changes at the menopause. There are also some differences in the way lesbian women approach changes in their sex lives, in that heterosexual women often believe or feel themselves more constrained by cultural ideas about menopause, gender and heterosexuality.[34]

Men, too, can be condemned to dissatisfaction and dysfunction by these narrow constraints. The novelist Howard Jacobson, in an article on sex and the older man, says he likes women who are the same age as he: 'Longevity is more beautiful to my eye. No look can rival for sexual excitement that of someone who has seen the world but still sees something he or she desires in you,' and 'Eroticism has nothing to do with youth and beauty but everything to do with intelligence and experience, spiced, preferably, with a little disappointment.' Jacobson believes that since the 1960s we have grown too literal minded about what constitutes sex (something that has much to do with the intervention of science, medicine and surveys, perhaps), that eroticism has been neglected in favour of athleticism, and that Viagra is a modern cruelty which fails to 'quicken' the mind.[35]

And what of late pregnancies which might result from all this sex? A WHO paper, 'Progress in Reproductive Health Research', astonishingly suggests that although women approaching the menopause can still become pregnant it 'is usually neither desired nor desirable' and so safe and effective contraception is needed. Leaving aside generalizations about what women might desire or whether medical opinion finds their desires 'desirable', the WHO recommends copper-bearing IUDs,[36] barrier methods,[37] combined oral contraceptives for women without contraindications[38] and sterilization. Methods of female sterilization include tubal resection, cautery and occlusion of the tube using bands or clips; over 40 per cent of couples over forty years of age in the UK have chosen one of these as a contraceptive option and a similar situation exists in many developed countries. The report says that half of all women in their early forties remain fertile and that, without contraception, the annual risk of pregnancy is about 10 per cent for women aged forty to forty-four, 2–3 per cent for those aged forty-five to forty-nine, and that for women over fifty it may not be zero. Official statistics in the UK show that 45 per cent of pregnancies among women over forty are terminated with legal abortion. Women in their forties have a maternal mortality rate four times that of women in their twenties and their risk of spontaneous abortion and perinatal mortality rates are double, at 26 per cent. The 'lifetime risk' of death from a pregnancy-related cause in the developing world is between one in fifteen and one in fifty, whereas the average lifetime risk in the developed world is between one in 4000 and one in 10,000. As the mortality rate rises with age, the menopause offers protection to women, especially in the developing world where it occurs usually five or more years earlier.[39]

Women who would like to delay having children need to know when they might enter the menopausal transition. They should ask their mothers, if they can, as the factors that determine age at menopause are about 85 per cent inherited. Studies are under way to discover which genes control the onset of the menopause and it is possible that in the future a blood test will scan a woman's genotype and reveal her expected age at menopause. Reproductive endocrinologists suspect that genes influence the size of the egg store present before birth and that the larger that store is, the later the menopause will occur. It is likely that genes also influence the rate at which eggs are used and, as more are wasted than are ovulated, drugs may be developed to delay eggs leaving 'the pool'. In February 2001 *Nature Genetics* magazine reported that the National Institute on Aging had proposed the possibility of a genetic trigger for early-onset menopause. The argument is that, although menopause is an age-related condition, all of the critical events that determine when the menopause will occur took place during foetal development and if more was understood about how tissues are formed, 'we might be able to prolong the function of cells and even regenerate tissues that are worn out'. By February 2006 researchers at the Medical University in Vienna had developed a test to predict the age at which a woman will enter the menopause and which could help 'career women' with their family planning.[40] The research concluded that the risk of early-onset menopause rested on many different factors, including age at first period, the number of children and miscarriages, a history of breast cancer as well as genetic variations, diet and smoking. Smokers, ex-smokers and passive smokers might reach the menopause up to two or three years earlier than those who have never smoked.[41] Research and development such as this can benefit young, infertile women and those who wish to delay pregnancy, and it could also mean the ability to prolong fertile life for older women – but with all the negative cultural connotations that elderly motherhood has come to involve.[42]

Real freedom to choose is extremely powerful and its consequences often surprising. The differences in power and control that men and women have over their socioeconomic circumstances – and so their mental and physical health, social position, status and treatment in society – impact directly on life experiences and events. It is no surprise that, according to the WHO, the most common mental disorders of depression and anxiety affect about one in three people, and predominantly women. It is argued that depression and anxiety are more persistent in women, but then they are more likely to be diagnosed and prescribed mood-altering psychotropic drugs than men, even when men present with identical symptoms. Although women are more likely to go to a GP whilst men are more likely to use inpatient care, the WHO maintains that women are more susceptible to depression and anxiety due to their multiple roles, gender discrimination and other associated factors which might exacerbate 'a sense of loss, inferiority, humiliation or entrapment'. In the *American Journal of Obstetrics and Gynecology* in 1971, Howard Osofsky and Robert Seidenberg expressed their opinion that

> It is no wonder that . . . women become depressed around the time of menopause; professionals and society have helped to ensure this reaction. At an age in life when a man is in the upswing of active social and professional growth, woman's service to the species is over. Professionals, including female experts, define the woman's role as one of mortification and uselessness.

Having sufficient autonomy and control over your own life, the material wherewithal to make choices and act upon them, and psychological support and knowledge are strong protections against depression. Studies have found 'no significant changes in anger, anxiety, depression, self-consciousness, or worry about the body between women observed from the time they were premenopausal to the time they had become postmenopausal'. Middle-aged

women today are less likely to be depressed than they were
ten years ago, and fewer menopausal women are depressed
than are women with young children.[43]

Anthropological studies show wide cultural differences in
experiences of depression. In Canada 82 per cent of women
agreed with the notion that 'women become depressed and
irritable at menopause', yet women in Rajput reported little
incidence of depression as at the menopause they could leave
off their veils, come out of seclusion and mix with men and a
wider social circle. In China, too, a greater respect for older
women means that menopausal symptoms, or their reporting as problematic, are rare. Women in transition between
traditional and modern lifestyles seem to suffer greater difficulties. Ethnic differences are recorded in the USA: Jewish
women have the highest rates of depression in menopause;
black women the lowest. One study of 2500 middle-aged
women in Massachusetts in the 1980s found that those who
had had a hysterectomy, with or without a bilateral
oophorectomy, had twice the rate of depression as those who
had a natural menopause, a significant finding in the light of
the popularity of the operation: nearly 30 per cent of women
there undergo hysterectomy, some 650,000 per year. The
researchers, perhaps unsurprisingly, reported that there was
a link between clinical depression and likelihood of surgery
and concluded that depression in middle-aged women was
mainly associated with events and circumstances unrelated
to hormonal changes. They also noted that most hormone
studies had relied on volunteers, 'a disproportionately large
number of whom have had hysterectomies'.[44]

Those arguing that menopausal depression caused
by endocrine changes exists believe it can be 'cured' by re-
establishing the hormonal balance with drug therapy, even

though the presumptuous medical notion of a right to adequate oestrogen from puberty to the grave is derived from the subjective and piecemeal information of self-selecting women. The psychiatrist Raj Persaud, speaking in London in 2005 at a Gresham College lecture on 'Depression: reality and myth', defined the menopause as a disease. Although it is, he said, a 'completely normal biological event' it 'attracts certain quite problematic medical symptoms, like osteoporosis, brittle bones, and a whole host of other things'. These 'things' should be treated, in his opinion, because it is not a question of whether it is normal or abnormal but, rather, of whether it is 'desirable', whether it 'leads to suffering'. His 'basic criterion of a disease' is suffering, and if medical technology can help it should be used. Persaud's 'basic criterion' could mean that life itself must be medically treated.

Persaud asserts that women are more prone to depression than are men, and that the reason for this is a 'very basic biological one', that women 'experience more quite clear biological life transitions' in puberty, pregnancy and menopause. Despite the obvious point that women are women by virtue of having these experiences, Persaud suggests that these events place enormous stress on them, far more than a man has to endure. It is a nonsense to compare the sexes on these terms and in so doing to place women in an invidiously helpless position, not unlike the Victorian notions of the feeble invalid weakened by her very femaleness, weak because of her sex. The 'stress on the female body' is a reason, Persaud believes, 'as to why women may be getting more depression than men'. Not only that, 'there's the biological turmoil' of her monthly periods, too. Concluding that 'no one really knows what is the bottom line answer', he admits his lack of real knowledge and so renders his spurious reasoning even less valid.

A connection between menopause and mental illness has a long history within the medical profession. In the nineteenth century depression experienced during or around the time of menopause was thought to cause insanity, and was categorized as a disease known as 'involutional melancholia'. This disease described the mental disturbances associated with the 'retrograde change which occurs in the body in old age, or in some organ when its permanent or temporary purpose has been fulfilled'. The influential German psychiatrist Emil Kraepelin (1856–1926), who developed a classification system for mental illness based on physiology rather than psychology, was the first to discuss the high incidence of an apparently common melancholia during the 'involutional period'. It was not until 1980 that the entry for this disease was removed from the third edition of the *Diagnostic and Statistical Manual of Mental Disorders*. Recent research has revealed that depressive illnesses are no different and no more likely to strike at menopause than at other times or stages of life. Women who are most susceptible to depression at menopause are those who have a history of depressive episodes. Depression should not be seen as a normal, natural or expected consequence of the menopause, and there is no evidence which shows an increase in depression among women at this time. The idea of the 'empty nest syndrome', which describes women whose children have left home and who experience a profound loss of purpose and identity, may exist but it is not a consequence of the menopause itself.

Despite a dearth of supporting evidence linking menopause and mental health there is still a drive to investigate the connection. A review of the available literature on the relationship between depression and natural menopause in the *British Medical Journal* (*BMJ*) in 1996 looked at ninety-four articles from over thirty years of research and found 'insufficient evidence to maintain that menopause causes depression'.[45] Another piece in the *BMJ* the same year found no evidence of researched formulated studies which attributed depression in middle-aged women directly to the menopause.[46] Epidemiological studies carried out in the 1980s on middle-aged women in North America and Europe found that psychosocial factors were the main predictors of depression during the menopausal period and that few changes related to depression could be attributed directly to the menopause. Research studies undertaken at Harvard Medical School on women who experienced depression during early-onset menopause came to similar conclusions, saying that, whilst 'there is an association between depression and premature menopause [. . .] it becomes apparent five, maybe fifteen years before actual menopause sets in', suggesting once again that there are reasons for depression in middle-aged women other than the menopause itself.[47]

The uncertainty around menopausal symptoms has led some researchers to argue for a psychological reason for mid-life changes rather than a biological, menopausal reason. The menopause accompanies these alterations rather than causes them. It's not a clearly marked event like menarche or pregnancy but a process that ranges over time, a decade or so. Women experience such varied 'symptoms' or sensations, and describe them so differently, that they are almost impossible to measure or gauge. How can we accurately measure the strength of libido and orgasm? Who is to say that a hot flush might not be pleasurable in some way to some women?[48]

Why do we even have a menopause? It's a peculiarity in biological terms and very nearly unique to humans. A woman at fifty is often in good physical condition, has accumulated useful experience and could live almost as many years after her menopause as she has done before it, so why should her reproductive function shut down? This biological behaviour appears to contradict the Darwinian principle of natural selection acting to maximize reproductive potential. Logic would have it that the reproductive system that operates the longest and most successfully should not be subject to decay and cessation but carry on throughout the natural lifespan. Yet only in humans do the eggs run out so early, despite our unusually long lives, the longest lifespan of any mammal.[49] There is no universal pattern of reproductive ageing, or senescence, in female vertebrates, rather there is a spectrum from the semelparous to the iteroparous: from creatures whose lives gear up to one burst of reproduction followed by death to those who reproduce in bouts throughout their lives. Women's long life history lies near the extreme iteroparous end of the spectrum with more reproductive opportunities and a slower senescence.[50]

Human longevity puts pressure on the body's maintenance system to work at higher levels but reduces its resources available for reproduction. That a woman's store of eggs runs out many years prior to the onset of general ageing is the evolutionary puzzle of the menopause – 'there is no reason related to general mechanisms of ageing for oozytes [eggs] not to last longer than fifty years'; human neurons, for example, can function for up to twice as long as this.[51] One plausible explanation is that an older mother, as she reaches the age of fifty or so, will start experiencing some of the adverse effects of natural ageing and if she then stops producing children she is more likely to enhance her genetic contribution to future generations by investing her energy and experience into caring for her later-born babies and grandchildren.[52] This is the 'grandmother hypothesis', first postulated in 1957 by G. L. Williams in his paper 'Evolution'. It argues that although, as a species, we do not stop reproducing particularly early in life we do survive longer; our late maturity, together with our long post-menopausal life, is distinctly human.[53] This theory, which reduces the female role to bearing and caring, still doesn't tell the whole story.

Despite our understanding of the biological mechanisms behind the menopause, it is still regarded as an evolutionary puzzle that females of some species have one while others don't (the two other species in which it occurs under natural conditions are killer whales and pilot whales). In theory there should be no selection for genes which promote survival past the end of reproduction. Humans are unique among primates because there is almost no overlap of reproductive generations. In populations where fertility occurs naturally, women on average have their first baby at nineteen and their last at thirty-eight. They stop breeding when the next generation begins to breed. The grandmother hypothesis is problematic in that 'data from natural fertility societies suggests that grandmothering benefits are too small to favour switching off reproduction by age fifty in order to help'. So while the theory explains why women continue to survive after the menopause, it can't explain why they stop breeding in the first place. Recent research now argues that the menopause is an adaptation to minimize reproductive competition between generations of females in the same family unit.[54] This makes sense in that, where mothers-in-law compete with their daughters-in-law, the latter would have the advantage. The mother-in-law, being related to the younger woman's children, shares an interest in her reproductive success, but it doesn't work in reverse. Indeed, in some societies, particularly in Africa and Asia, social law requires women to stop having children when their first grandchild is born.

It is often thought that, historically, women rarely lived long enough to go through their menopause, but this is to misunderstand average life expectancy. Even from the few medieval records that survive it is believed that as many as a quarter of the population reached menopausal age.[55] Average life expectancies were skewed by infant mortality rates – baby boys born in the UK in 1901 had only an 83 per cent chance of survival, girls an 86 per cent chance. For those of either sex born in 1951 there was a 97 per cent chance of surviving their first year. If you made it past puberty and childbirth you stood a very good chance of reaching old age, so the menopause was not at all an uncommon experience. Life expectancy for people born in Britain in 1851 was 40.2 years for men and 43.6 years for women. Fifty years later, in 1901, it was 50.3 years for men and 57.0 years for women. By 1951 it had risen rapidly to 77.3 years for men and 82.1 years for women. In America today overall life expectancy is 77.9 years. More and more women now spend longer in the post-menopausal period than ever before (at least in the West) yet seem to be more and more fearful. The fear of death is now seen to be associated with menopause, as it once was with pregnancy and childbirth.

There are some who argue that there is no such thing as 'the menopause', rather it is just a series of possible menopausal experiences which can happen within female life history as a consequence of ageing. Most studies of menopausal women have been carried out on Caucasian women from Western cultures. A study of nearly 15,000 women in America (Caucasian, African-American, Chinese, Japanese and Hispanic) aged 40–55 years in 1995–7, called the Study of Women's Health Across the Nation (SWAN),[56] found that there was a strong argument against a universal 'menopausal syndrome'. The type and number of menopausal symptoms, and the finding that they varied according to race and ethnicity, argued against the idea of a coherent syndrome. Compared with Caucasian women, all other racial/ethnic groups reported significantly fewer symptoms; perhaps unsurprisingly then, hormone use was highest among the Caucasian women and lowest among the African-American and Hispanic women. African-American women reported more vasomotor symptoms (hot flushes) and were more likely to have had a surgical menopause; Chinese and Japanese women in the groups were more likely to be peri-menopausal, differing the most from Caucasian women. Japanese women have lower rates of almost every suggested symptom than American and Canadian women of similar ages; a diet high in soy may account for their lower incidence of hot flushes. Individual and cultural influences illustrate just how complex the relationship is between bodily changes and the plethora of symptoms women say they experience.[57]

In Western culture the menopause is burdened with a terrible psychological weight because it has been written off as a pathological condition. In the 1970s feminists began to challenge the orthodox medical model of the menopause, viewing it instead as a positive transformation in life. Feminism positioned itself against the medicalization of the menopause, a process seen as a conspiracy by a gerontocracy, a male-dominated movement which relied upon the creation of a submissive female patient who could be treated with drugs. Feminism understands science, medicine, pharmaceutical companies and the media as being irrevocably gendered and promoting stereotypical male and female treatments. In her book *The Menopause Industry*, Sandra Coney argues that medicine discovered the sick mid-life woman and perpetrated the 'suspicion that some vile, vile, sinister disease process invades some body part, rendering bones in danger of imminent collapse, breasts about to erupt with mountainous lumps [and] vaginas wither up'.[58] If there are no obvious physical causes of illness then psychogenic ones label women neurotic in some specific way. The gulf between the description of menopause in medical texts – so unrelentingly negative, florid and quite frankly nausea-inducing – and the experience, is great. The answer is to liberate women from being labelled as physically wasting, psychologically impaired and socially worthless, whose only way back to health, desirability and validity, by remaining sexually capable to serve the needs of men, is 'a carload of hormones or a lobotomy'.[59] The early- to mid-twentieth-century focus on hormones and HRT distorted the picture of older women, their experiences and responses, in the name of progressive medical science, individual medics' careers, and the profits of pharmaceutical companies. Drug therapies came under suspicion and women began to voice their anger and dissatisfaction. To really understand the menopause, women's experiences of it have to be recorded, published and, not least, believed; this provides the balance to a historically male-dominated medical picture of the menopause where the ideology and language have been, too often, patronizing, alienating and subjugating.[60]

Gloria Steinem's famous article 'If men could menstruate', published in the October 1978 issue of *Ms* magazine, was written to challenge male-dominated cultural attitudes to the female body. Sceptical of Freud's notion of 'penis envy', she suggested that 'womb envy' was in play – that this unexposed organ with the power of giving birth held a terrible fascination for men. She turned a negative, menstruation, into a positive. If men could menstruate, Steinem posited, it would be an enviable, worthy, masculine event: they would boast about how long they bled and how much blood they could produce. It would be the 'beginning of manhood', celebrated with ritual, dinners, gifts and stag parties, and there would be a National Institute of Dysmenorrhea. Since men would be hormonally protected from heart attacks, medical funds would be diverted into cramps. Sanitary products would be free, surveys would prove that statistically men did better at sport during their periods. 'Men-struation' would mean that only men could occupy positions of power and that women were unclean because they *didn't* have a monthly purge. 'Lesbians would be said to fear blood and therefore life itself, though all they needed was a good menstruating man.' Women would be disconnected from the rhythm of the universe itself.

Steinem's arresting article was preceded by nearly a hundred years by a British surgeon, Thomas Spencer Wells, one of the few medical men to subvert the orthodox view:

> If we hold the mirror up to Nature, only changing the sex of the actors, the spectacle is not flattering. Fancy the reflected picture of a coterie of Marthas of the profession in conclave, promulgating the doctrine that most of the unmanageable maladies of men were to be traced to some morbid change in their genitals, founding societies for the discussion of them and hospitals for the cure of them, one of them sitting in her

consultation chair, with her little stove by her side and her irons all hot, searing every man as he passed before her . . . if too, we saw, in this magic mirror, ignorant boys being castrated almost impromptu, hundreds of emasculated beings moping about . . . should we not, to our shame, see ourselves as others see us? Should we not be bound . . . to denounce such follies as a personal degradation, a crime against society, and a dishonour to the profession?[61]

Science continues to be a powerful agent of the naturalization of women's place in society: determining gender roles by using arguments from nature and validating cultural ideas such as that a woman's place is in the home. But as notions of nature change over time so does the use of naturalization, so that, for example, educating women was opposed in the nineteenth century because of its alleged potential to corrupt a nature which understood them to be intellectually incapable, fit only for breeding. Later it became an economic argument wherein a woman's 'inferior' intelligence meant that the effort and resources put into her education were pointless. Female intellectuals went from being described as ridiculous and rebellious to just downright impossible, enabling Cesare Lombroso in *The Man of Genius* (1891) to strip them of their sex and maintain that 'There are no women of genius; the women of genius are men.' The oppressive aspects of the relationship between medicine and women have occurred at times of radical change – when there were calls for education, employment and votes for women, doctors were advising of their dreadful dangers. Conflating what is cultural with what is deemed natural became a common theme. Subjective supposition became objective fact. Culture was busy making the body and then understanding it as biological fact. Medicine has always been a question of cultural negotiation.[62]

The fantastically talented late Roy Porter, citing Ivan Illich and his theory of the 'medicalization of life', argued that the rapidly expanding medical establishment of the nineteenth century, faced with a healthier population of its own creation, found itself medicating normal life events, turning risks into diseases and treating trivial complaints with fancy procedures. Medicalization often meant stigmatization, and so it was with the medical account of the menopause.[63] The psychiatrist Thomas Szasz has suggested that physicians and especially psychiatrists have been over-zealous in attributing the word 'illness' to any and every detectable sign of malfunction, based on no matter what norm.[64] Its medicalization explains why the menopause is generally derided, feared and dismissed. The medical model and the language it uses have obscured the personal and social experience of the menopause. The phrase 'atrophy of genital tissues', though medically descriptive, smacks of decay and decline, loss and lack. 'Menopausal ovarian dysfunction' suggests that ovulating women are normal while those who no longer do so are abnormal. Just twenty years ago, when today's post-menopausal women may have begun to entertain thoughts of the menopause, articles by leading physicians in the field were still using terms such as 'exhausted', 'falter', 'demise', 'aberrations', 'distemper', 'wrinkled', sagging' and 'hunching'.[65] 'Many women', it was blithely suggested, 'are unable to cope and to adjust' to what the doctors, with unbearable archness, call '*charmes perdus*'. With language which couldn't get more archaic and euphemistic if it tried, they asserted that 'full-fashioned womanhood' had its own 'mystique' – language which simultaneously seeks to flatter and insult women with its nauseous sentimentality. Anything other than the cultural ideal of a sexually pert, compliant, fully functioning female is to be despised and avoided at all costs. It will come as no surprise that the authors are leading proponents of thaumaturgic hormone replacement therapy which will maintain a woman's sexual availability and 'delay the inevitable'. The implication is that women are somehow victims of their bodies, that they have no control over them or, in effect, themselves.

Despite challenges to medical orthodoxy, late-twentieth-century descriptions of the menopause mirror those of fifty years ago. In 1945 the psychoanalyst Helen Deutsch, in her book *The Psychology of Women*, referred to the menopause as a 'partial death' in which 'everything [a woman] acquired during puberty is now lost piece by piece; with the lapse of the reproductive service, her beauty vanishes, and usually the warm, vital flow of feminine emotional life as well'. Nearly fifty years later, in 1992, Germaine Greer suggested in *The Change* that the menopause 'is a time for mourning . . . the menopausal woman should be allowed her quiet time and her melancholy'.[66] Our understanding of the menopause depends on who is doing the talking, the language they are using, the audience, the time, place and context; it is chronology and interpretation.

The origin of the modern menopause reaches as far back as Greek and Roman medical thought and is entrenched in deep-seated ideas of the innate sickness of women, of deformity and lack. In 1987 Dr Robert Greenblatt was preaching the same theory of lack and decay, acknowledging the added touch of nineteenth-century madness: 'before the advent of modern endocrinology, the vexations of this phase of a woman's life were considered a hysteroneurosis'; now she is in 'an oestrogen-deprivation state'. In many ways hormonal explanations have come to dominate contemporary thought and an endocrinological narrative of menopause has led to the conclusion that menopausal women should be manipulated with drugs. But the backlash has begun. It can clearly be seen that the many cultural meanings of the menopause are chaotic and unclear because its origins lie in changing perceptions and knowledge, rather than in a determined biology.

2

BAD BLOOD AND BEASTS

What is woman? Disease, says Hippocrates.

Horatio Storer (1830–1922), gynaecologist and president of
the American Medical Association

Greek and Roman physicians knew that women were inferior creatures — different, weak, whorish, irrational, prone
to sickness and in constant need of supervision. They were
inherently pathological, condemned by medicine at its very
outset, and of interest primarily because of their reproductive
system. Once this had ceased, at their climacteric, they stood
alone at the gateway to death. This classical definition of
women's bodies underpins modern Western medical thought
about women. It provided the basis for all the prejudices,
cruelties, experiments, misapprehensions and misguided
treatments which crowded medical texts and practices for
centuries afterwards.

In the classical system the human body was subject to particular periods or eras dictated by considerable and general

changes, and these climacteric periods occurred in multiples of seven years. The term 'climacteric' comes from the Greek, meaning a step of a stair or rung of a ladder. The 'grand climacteric' is the term commonly applied today to the period of female menopause which the Greeks placed in the forty-ninth year; it came into English through Philemon Holland's translation of Pliny in 1601. The term 'menopause' is from the Greek too – the prefix 'men' originates in the Greek for month, in the plural it meant the menses or monthly periods of women, and 'menopause' is the cessation of the menses.[1] If the medical writers did not specifically describe the menopause they did acknowledge its existence. Menarche differentiated women from men and menstruation defined a female body as weak and in need of supervision, supporting the idea of a woman's subordinate and restricted role. However, menopause brought women closer in ideal to the male body, and so did not require specialized medical knowledge.

All aetiology, symptoms and treatments of menstruation described women as lesser creatures. The philosopher Aristotle (384–322 BC) believed that the apparent abundance of menstrual blood compared with seminal fluid underpinned the ascendancy of the male of almost every species, and this was all the more obvious in humankind.[2] Life, he thought, is dependent on heat and moisture and over a lifespan an animal uses up its innate heat, becoming colder and drier and nearer to death. The menopause fitted in well with this model.[3] The lack of any truly dire menopausal effects combined with the older woman's apparent similarity to the Greek male ideal meant that there was no need for a gynaecological explanation of how a body of this sort might work. Medicine was unsure whether women had diseases peculiar to their sex or whether they suffered from the same conditions as men, only requiring a separate specialism, gynaecology, for their different organs.[4]

To Hippocrates (460–370 BC), said to be so proficient in the healing arts that he reduced the number of shades in Hades, the cessation of bleeding meant the reassimilation of the unruly female body with the male, knowable and supposedly more orderly body.[5] These ideas were inherited by Galen of Pergamum (AD 129–c. 216), who was practising in Rome. Galen was the most influential of physicians in later antiquity, whose work was still central to Western medicine in the eighteenth century.[6] He believed women to be imperfect and mutilated examples of the ideal male form who, when their periods stopped, became less feminine and more 'manly-hearted'. These notions, of course, speak of the threat of female power and the challenge to male dominance, and they have fostered a constant concern and source of ambivalence and anxiety.

Medical texts gave a relentlessly male version of women's bodies, emotions, functions, capacities and daily lives, defining woman as being what man was not, in both a confrontational and a complementary way. The most obvious difference between men and women was their reproductive roles and women were solely understood by physicians as child bearers.[7] Their 'perpetual infirmities' are described in the *Hippocratic Corpus*, a collection of medical treatises probably assembled in the third or second century BC at Alexandria. The Hippocratic authors were practising physicians who wrote their theses intending to improve therapies and increase custom while pursuing their academic interest in medical knowledge. Ten of the sixty or so treatises in the *Corpus* are gynaecological in nature.[8] The female body was considered very vulnerable during the period from menarche to menopause; her reproductive years were biologically threatening. The Greek word '*gynē*' is used both for woman and for wife, laying emphasis on the positive, domesticated values of reproductive womanhood. Negative values were attributed to the unmarried, widowed and the post-menopausal, no longer bearing children. The *Hippocratic Corpus* had established female physical 'norms' and made a distinction between the 'womb-woman' and those 'outside the logic of regeneration', the necessarily illogical beings of the pre-pubescent and the post-menopausal.[9] Many priestesshoods seem to have been reserved for post-menopausal women. Plutarch says that the Pythia was the only woman allowed in the temple at Delphi and that she had to be past fifty years old.[10]

The Hippocratic tracts emphasized that the body was inherently unstable, liable to disease, hard to diagnose and often impossible to cure. The four humours – black bile, yellow bile, phlegm and blood – considered part of the essential make-up of humans, were extended to cover the four elements (earth, air, water and fire), the four seasons, the four qualities (hot, cold, wet and dry), the four ages of man, and the four mental states or temperaments. Health and disease were dependent on the balance or imbalance of the elements, seen as the building blocks of the body and of the universe, of the fluids or 'humours', of 'powers' (hot and cold, sweet and sour) and of 'fluxes' that caused harm by settling in a wrong place. Seasonal changes, heredity and the patient's environment also affected the balance of health. This system provided a rationale for understanding the individual in sickness and in health, and against the wider cosmos, and it held sway for centuries.[11] Women's bodies were deemed to be cold

and wet and those of men to be warm and dry, and whereas
the male sweats to rid himself of impurities and 'superfluous
humours', the female bleeds.[12]

The *Corpus* regarded the reproductive functions of the
female body as pathological conditions requiring treatment,
yet this state of sickness was understood as being wholly natural, for it was completely wrong for women to develop
masculine characteristics.[13] Women were not simply sub-
standard to men but were quite different creatures, so the
Corpus did not need to construct a correspondence between
all male and female body parts as Aristotle did. As women's
legal, social and economic lives began to expand in the
Hellenistic period (*c.* 323 BC to roughly the end of the first
century BC), the Aristotelian model of female physiology was
displacing the traditional Hippocratic view among practising physicians and it used 'scientific' theory to argue for the
natural subordination of women to men. Women were inferior but their 'otherness' meant that their bodies could be
defined more by their own characteristics and parameters.[14]
They lacked male perfection of mind and body and were
therefore nearer to beasts, and their reproductive organs
were considered to be the most animal-like in their bodies,
even to the extent of having horns. For Plato the uterus was
an animal with its own sense of smell, a living creature longing to bear children which wandered about the body leaving
disease and disorder in its wake.[15] As animalistic 'potential
whores . . . slaves to their emotions, of which only men can
be a master', women's lack of self-control and consequent
fierce licentiousness were a force of 'undisciplined evil' which
had to be domesticated so that they could reproduce in the
male-structured society.

There was a strong correlation between good health and

menstruation, and to promote this regular purge women were prescribed alterations in their diet, vapour baths, fumigations, pessaries and fomentations.[16] Galen thought that the well-purged woman would be unaffected by podagra (gout), arthritis, pleuritis, peripneumonia, epilepsia, apoplexia, apnoea (breathlessness), phrentis (brain fever), lethargos, spasmos, tromos (dread), tetanus, melancholia, mania, spitting and vomiting blood, kephalaia, synanchic suffocation and any other major and serious disease, meaning that those whose menses were suppressed or had ceased might suffer many of these terrible ills. He developed an argument from nature for the physician's use of phlebotomy – bloodletting – around menstruation in *On Venesection against Erasistratus*:

> Does she [nature] not evacuate all women every month, by pouring forth the surfeit of the blood? For it is necessary, I think, that the female genus, who stays at home, neither leading a life of hard work nor coming into contact with direct sunlight, and because of both these things generating excess, should have a natural remedy – the evacuation of excess . . . If you knew what great benefits the female genus enjoys as a result of this evacuation, and how she is harmed if not purged, I don't know how you could still hesitate and not eagerly evacuate surplus blood by all means.[17]

Galen naturalized women's social role by aligning this with female physical characteristics of the soul: in his *Usefulness of the Parts* he states that a man is 'more august, especially as he grows older', whilst about women he decrees that 'this animal does not have an august character as the man has and so does not need an august form'. He repeats many times throughout the work that 'nature makes the form of the body appropriate to the characteristics of the soul . . . for the most part women stay at home'. In *Affected Places* he describes the suffocation of the womb, an early understanding of hysteria brought on by the travelling womb violently compressing other vital organs into a narrow space and causing choking, loss of breathing, speech and sensibility.[18] He elaborated on the way this plight affected the older, deprived woman:

> It is generally agreed that this affection occurs, for the most part, in widows, and especially when those who previously used to menstruate and bear children well, and who were accustomed to sexual intercourse with men, are deprived of all these things. And so, what more persuasive conclusion could be drawn from these things than that these so-called uterine dispositions occur in women because of the stoppage of the menses . . . whether [the dispositions] happen to be apnoic, suffocatory, or convulsive?[19]

Still, scant attention was paid to the menopause and post-menopause, with little attempt to explain in detail how or why a woman's body ceased to bleed regularly, nor did there seem much awareness of the discomforts that women might suffer around this time. The Hippocratics had older women among their clientele, referring to 'elderly' female patients and reporting that they were dry, their wombs were empty and light, and they had less blood than younger women, presumably because they had ceased to menstruate. The Hippocratics probably – and correctly – believed that post-menopausal women had ceased to produce blood rather than it having become trapped in the body, as later physicians assumed. In Western society today the emphasis on female change is the other way around so that menarche seems to carry few biological threats whilst menopause is laden with disorders and suffering – perhaps because youth is idolized and age is devalued.[20]

Little is known about how women saw the world they inhabited and their voices are largely silent in these classical writings. Their traces can be discerned only through the actions, the words and the laws of men. Many of these traces define women as 'near-slaves, or as perpetual mirrors' whose 'greatest glory . . . is to be least talked about by men'. Pliny, remarking on female vanity, argued that women were characterized by a great concern for their appearance and that the vast majority of cosmetic recipes were specifically labelled for women. Celsus complained that 'to treat pimples, spots, and freckles is almost absurd'. Women existed here as objects of knowledge attracting male criticism, but there is very little on their own actual experiences. Where the works of female medical authorities were known – those of Salpe, Elephantis, Lais, and others – deep suspicion surrounded them. Their expertise in gynaecology could not overcome their gender or poor social status. Pliny recorded traditional female knowledge but took care to qualify it, warning that 'it is better not to believe them' and that some of their skills were used not only by midwives but also by prostitutes. It is probably true that women's medical activity continued unaffected by the development of all this medical literature. It was men who acted in the world and required this knowledge to act, the male being the measure of the world; women did not give definition or meaning but were fashioned in their realization.[21]

Ancient philosophical traditions eventually merged with

Judeo-Christian thought. Saint Augustine (AD 354–430), one of the most significant thinkers in the development of Christianity, argued in his *Confessions* that, although in her mind and intelligence a woman is equal to man, it is her biological sexual role which renders her resolutely subordinate. Although Augustine's ideas were humane in intent they are unremittingly oppressive in effect, and because he was one of the most influential figures of medieval philosophy his authority and thought came to exert a pervasive and enduring influence well into the modern period. Female inferiority and subordination were supported most notably by the Genesis narrative of Eve's derivation from Adam's rib and her seduction by the serpent, which seemed to many early Christian writers to be a watertight rationale for defining women and resisting their freedoms.[22]

The menopause is bound up with the presence or absence of blood. The deep, visceral symbolism of blood, that vital fluid, its preciousness, its perceived susceptibility to corruption, has always generated a flood of intellectual and cultural responses. Bleeding was regarded from ancient times as both good and bad (as with the old rhyme for little girls, when it is good, it is very, very good and when it is bad, it is horrid). The presence of menstrual blood was generally seen as a good thing as, whilst it was in essence foul and poisonous, its regular purging flow purified the body. The absence of blood at the menopause was a terrible negative, as the poison was thought to be retained and to wreak havoc in the body; its suppression could not be underestimated.

The texts of Leviticus construed menstruating women as polluted and polluting and placed many restrictions on women's behaviour; Isaiah 30:22 says that the coverings of images should be cast away 'as a menstruous cloth', and

Ezekiel 18:18 notes that 'one of the properties of a good man [is] not to lie with a menstruous woman'.[23] The basis of Jewish menstrual laws is found in chapter 15 of Leviticus. The Hebrew term used for menstruation is '*niddah*', from the root *ndh* which means 'separation' usually because of impurity, and is connected to the root *ndd*, which means 'to make distant'. It came to be used as a metaphorical expression for sin and impurity in general. Leviticus 20:21 mentions the sin of adultery or incest with one's brother's wife and uses the word '*niddah*', and in other biblical texts the term refers to abominable acts or status, especially sexual sins and idolatry. This separation limited and determined women's public and private lives if they were of child-bearing age. In public a menstruating woman could not enter the Temple, and in private she could not touch the food or objects which required a ritual state of purity. Touching a menstruating woman made one impure until sunset, as did touching whatever she sat or lay down on. If contaminated, a man would bathe and wash his clothes. Sex transferred the woman's entire seven days of impurity to the man, as well as the power to contaminate others (Lev. 15:24).[24]

In sixth-century Byzantium, Aëtius Amidenus, physician to Justinian I, discussed the age at which a woman might stop bleeding in his work *Tetrabiblos*, saying: 'The menses do not cease before the thirty-fifth year nor appear after the fiftieth; rarely some menstruate until the sixtieth year. Those who are very fat cease early.'[25] These estimates treat the menopause as a transitional period which might happen at any time over a period of up to twenty-five or thirty years, sometimes more on rare occasions, depending on the individual woman's physiology and environment. The most frequently cited age at menopause was fifty years, just as it is today, and ages of over fifty were more commonly suggested than ages below that. Paulus Aegineta, a seventh-century medical compiler, agreed: 'Some cease menstruating around the fiftieth year, rarely some [continue] until the sixtieth, but in some, especially those who are very fat, the menses begin to cease from the thirty-fifth year.' In Europe the medical school at Salerno, Italy, became a centre for knowledge and learning from the tenth century onwards and Trotula di Ruggiero wrote a two-part medical treatise here, *De Egretudinibus Mulierum* ('Trotula Major') and *De Ornamentis Mulierum* ('Trotula Minor'). Generally attributed to the late eleventh century, it became immensely popular in England – there are eighteen separate medieval manuscripts of it in Oxford alone. The first work contains a passage on menarche and menopause:

> This purge occurs in women around the fifteenth year (or a little earlier or later), according to their greater or lesser degree of heat or cold; and it lasts until the fiftieth year if the woman is thin; until sixty or fifty-five if she is moist; until thirty-five in the moderately fat.

In *c.* 1160–70 a compilation of Salernitan medical texts, *De Aegritudinum Curatione*, included the work of the physician John Platearius the Younger, who wrote, 'The retention [of the menses] is natural in old age just as it is contrary to nature from the fifteenth year up to the sixtieth year.' Interestingly, he is emphatic in saying that, 'since retention of the menses does not occur after sixty years [of age], it is not *curable*'. Thomas of Cantimpre, who produced an ency-clopaedic work, *De Natura Rerum*, between 1228 and 1244, maintained that 'a woman conceives clear up to the fiftieth year'; Gilbert Angelicus' *Compendium Medicinae*, c. 1230–40, agrees that 'the menses are naturally retained below the twelfth year and above the fiftieth'; and Bartholomeus Angelicus, in his *De Rerum Proprietatibus*, c. 1240, suggests that retention of the menses was a cause for concern 'generally from the fourteenth up to the fiftieth year', but not beyond that. A Fellow of Merton College, Oxford, John of Gaddesden, who wrote the *Rosa Medicinae* or *Rosa Anglica* between 1305 and 1317, said that 'the menses are withheld naturally until the twelve or fourteenth years and after fifty, although in some cases they cease earlier, at thirty-five, forty, or forty-five, according to the various natures of the women'.[26] At least one historian believes that these estimates of age at menopause are perhaps a little credulous because, if accepted, 'it still leaves us with a fairly generalized view of the possible ages in question; the menopause figures especially are so wide-ranging as to invite wholesale rejection'.[27] But these medieval physicians are all describing a transitional phenomenon that fits into the natural order of the physical world, in tune with classical medical teaching. The menopause, or retention of bleeding, is wide-ranging and may occur at any time over a period of up to thirty years depending on the individual woman, and it needs no cure because it is not an illness.

Although some definitions of the menopause were fairly loose, the belief that ordinarily flowing menstrual blood was a foul excretion was regularly repeated. The French medieval work *Secrets des dames* explained to its readers that 'whosoever were to take a hair from the pubis of a woman and mix it with menses and then put it in a dung-heap, would at the end of the year find wicked venomous beasts'. This misogynistic recipe of hair, blood and fertile filth is an example of the myth of poisonous blood, widespread from the end of the thirteenth century. It had a toxic hangover which infected later centuries, apparent in the case-books of physicians and astrologers and in the diaries of some men who commented on their wives' and mistresses' menstrual experiences. In the privacy of their diaries men such as Samuel Pepys and Ralph Josselin used the straightforward dismissive 'them' or 'those' to describe periods, certainly nothing to do with 'us'.[28] Sir William Monson's wife, who consulted Simon Forman in 1597, when she had 'not her course and the menstrual blood runneth to her head' was, he recorded, 'much subject to melancholy and full of fancies . . . And she thinks the devil doth tempt her to do evil to herself.'[29] The language commonly used to refer to periods was either pragmatic, such as 'flowers', 'terms', 'courses' and 'months', or expressions of weakness, such as 'sickness', 'monthly disease' and 'monthly infirmity'.[30] Medical writers used Latin or Greek words to describe menstruation, such as *menstris*, *menses* or *catamenia*, general terms such as 'monthly evacuations' and 'natural purgations', and also meaningfully weighted terms like 'the time of your wonted grief' and 'those Evacuations of the weaker Sex'.

The cathartic purging of a venomous discharge is one thing, whilst cessation of bleeding and the retention of bloody poisons is another. A woman's lack of natural heat (women, remember, were cold and wet whilst men were warm and dry) and her allegedly less active life hampered her body in its task of shedding the potentially harmful residues of excess blood and other unnecessary fluids. A theory of fermentation and effervescence of the blood was popular, wherein the good matter was separated from the bad as it 'flings up to the Surface a sort of Scum abounding with Air, which is call'd the *Flowers*', and it explained why women 'often [became] sick with the cessation of their monthlies'. Daniel Duncan, in his *Chymie Naturelle* (1687), described how the 'filter of the uterus' weakened with age and was unable to shed the corrupt humours which languished 'like a dead sea' with 'no flux and reflux'. A woman in this condition might come to resemble 'the sick who are close to death'.

Menstrual blood, believed corrupt, 'vitiated and almost sick', had the power to kill plants, caterpillars and insects. It could turn mirrors blind, and cause infertility, miscarriage, rabies and madness. In his work *De Insomniis*, Aristotle had stated that women were 'monsters' and a menstruating woman would stain any mirror she looked at with a bloody cloud.[31] The Jacobean dramatist and poet Barnabe Barnes (1568–1609), fourth son of the Bishop of Durham, insulted the soul of Pope Alexander VI with a menstrual simile when the Devil denounced Alexander, declaring:

Thy soule foule beast is like a menstruous cloath,
Polluted with unpardonable sinnes.

Nicolas Fontaine believed that menstrual blood was 'in its own nature filthy, and dreggish'; it could

beget vapours which doe not onely assault the braine, but they oppresse the heart also . . . for when a gloomy and black vapour ascends to the braine, the principall parts, and their instruments are depraved, and the animal spirit, which is the chiefest instrument of the soule . . . is rendered darke, and obscure . . . they groane, they lament, anon againe they laugh . . . they turne, vary and alter their gestures . . . [they] have a conceit they are talking with Angels, sometimes they murmur, sometimes they sing . . . a thousand, several, ridiculous, and antick behaviours.[32]

Albertus Magnus's *Book of Secrets* (*De secretis mulierum: or, The Mysteries of Human Generation Fully Revealed*, 1725) warned that the eyes of a child in the cradle would be damaged if a woman who had ceased to menstruate should look at it.[33] She was dangerous, as well as depressed and mad. With 'the *monstrous* bloud detained in great abundance', a woman's body was considered frighteningly endangered and could succumb to chronic languor, dropsy, epilepsy, consumption, the potent threat of cancer of the uterus or breast and even sudden death.[34] Galen had linked breast cancer to the cessation of menses, assuming that blood that had once flowed freely would stagnate within the body and poison it. He believed that, if quickly diagnosed, the cancer could be cured by purging the body of the excess black bile which caused it. A cancer, wrote Fontaine, 'is an uneven, blewish swelling with paine, and filthy to behold' and, if ulcerated, it produced 'sordid lips, from whence issueth a black corruption, unsavoury and stinking'. Care was palliative, a good diet and rest and an avoidance of melancholy foods; surgery was out because, 'in regard of the consent which it hath with the braine [she] would presently perish'.[35]

The odd physician did challenge the idea that menstrual blood was a foul poison. In 1582 Jean Liébault argued that 'in itself [it] does no harm to the woman's body, except by its mere quantity'. Woman, he thought, produced more blood than she needed so that when she became pregnant it could nourish the foetus, and if she didn't her body would simply shed it. If this were the case then the menopause could be seen as a natural, innocuous process whereby the quantity of blood diminished as the woman aged. Nearly 200 years later, in 1771, Henry Manning gave his views on the 'ill-grounded prejudices' surrounding menstrual blood, laying them firmly at the feet of rabbis, noting that in hotter climes blood 'detained for some time among the folds of the vagina, must necessarily acquire an higher degree of acrimony than in more temperate climes' and, 'as commerce with women in that situation was sometimes observed to produce certain inconveniences to the other sex, it was expressly forbidden by the law of Moses'. Women were to perform specific ablutions to be cleansed before 'renewing the freedoms of the conjugal state' and

> Jewish priests, mistaking the genuine sense of their legislator, interpreted these necessary precautions into an insinuation of some inherent malignity . . . and by degrees, superstition, to which they were naturally much addicted, supplied a thousand chimeras to confirm their opinion. By this means, and the carelessness of succeeding times . . . the menstrual blood came at length to be universally stigmatised as a poisonous recrement.[36]

Motherwort, or mugwort, was a constantly used remedy for relieving suppression of the menses and promoting bleeding. *Bancke's Herbal* (1525) says that

> This herb in Latin is called Artemisia, and is hot and dry in the third degree [it] cleanseth the mother (uterus) and maketh a woman to have her flowers (menses), and it destroyeth emerods in this manner. First they must be gathered; then take powder of motherwort and horehound together, and strew it on the paps (swellings). Also, if a child

be dead in the mother's womb, take motherwort and stamp
it small and make a plaster thereof, and lay it to her womb all
cold, and with the grace of God she shall have deliverance
without peril.[37]

Another all-round, sure-fire remedy for women's discomfort and distress was a good orgasm. Nicholas Culpeper's
Practice of Physic (1678) advised that the 'genital Parts should be
by a cunning Midwife so handled and rubbed as to cause an
evacuation', but this being a possibly dubious activity, 'it may
suffice whilst the patient is in her bath to rub her belly in the
Region of the Womb'. This excellent advice ran through
eight printings and a total of 15,000 copies. In his work *The
Womans Doctour* (1652), Nicolas Fontaine expressed the view
that 'Wives are more healthfull than Widowes, or Virgins,
because they are refreshed with the man's seed.' These
women could ejaculate and the causes of their 'evil' would
be banished with their fluids. Those who were not so
refreshed, especially the widows, could have their 'spermat-
ick humour' diminished by 'the hand of a skilfull midwife,
and a convenient oyntment'. Fontaine had an astute eye on
his market, describing his remedies as 'Being Safe in the
Composition, Pleasant in the Use, Effectuall in the
Operation, Cheap in the Price'. And, luckily for his profits,
the diseases he described were common to all women:
widows and wives, barren and fruitful, and proceeded from
'stoppage of the courses'. Women, he stated,

> were made to stay at home, and to looke after Household
> employments, and because such business is accompanied
> with much ease, without any vehement stirrings of the body,
> therefore hath Nature assigned them their monthly Courses,

that by the benefit of those evacuations, the feculent and
corrupt bloud might be purified, which otherwise, as being
the purest part of the bloud, would turne to rank poison,
should it remain in the body and putrifie.[38]

According to Felix Platter, in 1656, God had designed the
menopause so that women would be fertile for a limited time
only, so preventing mankind from increasing to such numbers that the earth would be unable to support and nourish
everyone. 'Levinus Lemnius', however, in his volumes of *The
secret miracles of nature: in four books: learnedly and moderately treating of
generation, and the parts thereof* . . . (1658), expressly linked
women's fertility with the operation of 'the soul, and its
immortality'. Thomas Cogan's *Haven of Health* (1584), Helkiah
Crooke's *Mikrokosmographia* (1631), John Freind's *Emmenologia*
(1703), John Astruc's *Treatise on all the Diseases Incident to Women*
(1740) and John Anderson's *Medical Remarks on Natural,
Spontaneous and Artificial Evacuation* (1787) all agreed that the
process usually began at the '*second Septenary*, and terminated at
the *seventh*, or the square of the number Seven'. John Graunt's
demographic calculations of 1662 stated that women bred
from either sixteen to forty years, or twenty to forty-four,
and that if menarche was delayed so was menopause. It was a
natural phenomenon commonly experienced and Gregory
King, in his study of population by age, *Natural and Political
Observations* (1696), showed a large number of women still alive
at over sixty years old, practically all of whom would have
been post-menopausal.

There were plenty of popular explanations of the workings
of the female body for the public audience too. The anonymous, infamously lewd and extremely popular *Aristotle's
Master-Piece: or, The Secrets of Generation Displayed in all the Parts*

thereof, published in London in 1694, began in the first chapter to uncover the female body:

> At fourteen years of age, commonly, the *Menses* in Virgins begin to flow, and then they are capable of conceiving, and so continue generally to Forty-four; at what time for the most part, they are no longer capable of Generation, unless such as are exceeding healthfull, strong of Body, and have used themselves to Temperance, who have appear'd to be deliver'd of Children till Fifty five years; but such Prodigies rarely happen, altho' the *Menses* continue longer in some Women than in others; but many time such Eflux proceeds not from any natural cause, but by reason of some violent straining, or other violence, and doth oft endanger the Life of the Party: And therefore young Men that Marry Women surmounting the Age aforesaid, if they expect Children, unless by Miracle, must labour against the Wind: Though if an Old Man, that is not worn out by Diseases and Incontinence, Marry a brisk lively Lass, there is hopes even to Threescore and Ten, and some that are exceeding lusty, till Fourscore.

Aristotle's Compleat Master-Piece (1749) gave the established humoural explanation of menopause when answering the puzzle of 'why a Woman is sooner barren than a Man?': the 'natural Heat, which is the Cause of Generation, is more predominant in Men than Women, for the monthly Purgations of Women shew them to be more moist than Men, and so does also the Softness of their Bodies'. The enormously popular sequel to this work, *Aristotle's Book of Problems*, contained 'divers Questions and Answers, touching the state of Man's Body', and the thirtieth edition, published in London in 1776, asked:

Q. For what reason do they leave at about fifty?
A. '. . . nature is weak in them, and therefore they cannot expel them by reason of weakness . . . this makes them troubled with coughs and other infirmities. Men should refrain their use at those times.'

Older women were thought to become too frail to bleed, to succumb to debilitating sicknesses, and should be left alone – perhaps they might even affect or infect men. At any rate, some physicians thought sex should be denied. But William Gouge (1578–1653) argued in his work *Of Domesticall Duties* (1622) that although procreation was one purpose, or 'end', of marriage it was not the only one and sexual 'duty' was to be rendered to 'wives [who] have left bearing'.[39]

Only occasionally did menopause surface in women's common-place books from this period, where everyday remedies and potions were routinely recorded. This lack of material or treatments should not be taken to mean that some women didn't suffer menopausal discomfort, but most would have treated their own ailments. One of the first English gynaecological handbooks, written by a woman, covered menopause 'because there are many women who have numerous diverse illnesses – some of them almost fatal'. Following classical teaching the book defined women as having 'less heat in their bodies than men and . . . more moisture because of lack of heat that would dry their moisture and their humors' but, nevertheless, they have 'bleeding which makes their bodies clean and whole from sickness. And they have such purgations from the age of twelve to fifty.'[40] These bloody purgations, it continues, 'come out of the veins that are in the uterus that is called the "mother" . . . [which is] a skin in which the child is enclosed in his mother's womb'. Many of the sicknesses that women suffered from were thought to come from the ailments of this 'mother' and were more often than not 'concerned with the stopping of the blood that they should have in their purgation and be purged of'. The cessation of bleeding was thought to 'occur in various ways and for various reasons: because of the heat or the cold of the uterus or the heat or the cold of the humours that are enclosed inside the uterus, or excessive dryness of their complexion, or being awake too much, thinking too much, being too angry or too sad, or eating too little'. There might be 'aching and suffering', heaviness, haemorrhoids, heart disease, fainting, dizziness, and a 'desire to consort with men'.

Various remedies are recommended, such as vicarious bloodletting in other places on the body to get rid of the blood that has not been expelled. The veins of the big toe were popular – 'cut one day on one big toe then the other the next'; also cuts on the legs below the calf, both in front and behind. It suggests cupping, a treatment where heated cups are placed on the skin to create a vacuum and stimulate blood flow, 'under the nipples and also under the kidneys at the back'. Baths made from herbs were recommended, 'to open the veins of the uterus', with polypody, aurel leaves, ivy, savin, madder, oreganom, rosemary, cumin, asphodel, fennel, Artemisia, calamint, hyssop, wilde thyme and catmint. 'Let her sit on a hollow stool', the author writes, 'over these herbs when they are well boiled and hot' and bathe once a week in the herbal bath.[41]

St Hildegarde of Bingen produced a compendium of natural healing methods, *Liber Simplicis Medicinae*, in twelfth-century Germany, which gives a good idea of the remedies known and tested for generations by women healers. She lists the healing properties of 213 varieties of plants and fifty-five trees, plus dozens of mineral and animal derivatives, and effective painkillers, digestive aids and anti-inflammatory agents, including ergot for labour pains – this when the Church held that pain at childbirth was an imperative as punishment for Eve's original sin. Ergot derivatives are still used today to hasten labour and recovery from childbirth. Belladonna is also still used as an anti-spasmodic, to inhibit intense contractions when miscarriage is threatened. Digitalis is used now for heart disease and was said to have been discovered by an English 'witch'.[42] Hildegarde was a 'theologian, scientist and physician' with a reputation as a mystic. She lived in religious houses from the age of eight, founded the Rupertsberg Convent near Bingen in 1147, and lived there until she died in her early eighties in 1179. She would have had ample opportunity to observe the characteristics of menopause and treat the Benedictine nuns in her care. In Book II of her work *Causae et Curae*, in the section *De menstruo*, Hilegarde wrote that 'in women the menses are lacking after the fiftieth year, except in those who are healthy and strong, as in those the menses continue clear up to the seventieth year'. Further on, in *De menstrui defectu*, she says

the menses cease in women . . . when the uterus begins to be enfolded and to contract, so that they are no longer able to conceive. Sometimes it rarely happens that the occasional woman from any superfluity whatsoever with difficulty conceives a single time even up to the eightieth year. In the child, nevertheless, some defect arises sometimes, just as happens often in those who, being soft, young girls under their twentieth year, conceive and deliver in that tenderest age.[43]

The Book of Margery Kempe (c. 1423–c. 1438) reveals a knowledge of medicine derived from the Greek classics and intended for the 'good housewife' who might be more effective in treating her family than many an expensive physician or surgeon. Kempe was born in c. 1373 in the port town of King's Lynn, Norfolk, the daughter of the merchant John Brunham. She married when she was about twenty years old and had fourteen children. After what was described as a period of insanity following continuous childbirth, from her early forties to her sixties she travelled in England, in Europe, to the Holy Land and to Prussia – an extraordinary thing to do then, and even now quite an undertaking. Post-menopausal, free from society's expectations of her as wife and mother, and as likely mistress of her own funds, she took off overseas.[44]

Kempe's descriptions of her spiritual and psychological experiences bordered on what some scholars have chosen to see as madness. This ever-present ambivalence towards the lives of older women has led some historians to argue that a fear of women's sexuality contributed to the concepts of heresy and witchcraft. This punitive repression was a precursor to cultural nervousness about older women with their wandering wombs and their dangerously independent 'lustiness'. The threats posed by the post-fertile, 'manly-hearted' woman who could indulge in sex without fear of pregnancy, who had power, but remained different and irrational all served to exclude and castrate mid-life women no longer weighed down by children, menstruation and pregnancy. They were frighteningly free to join in with men and take, or at the very least want, to share their power. Rationality and self-control were identified as masculine virtues, as opposed to the animality, lust and unreason of women; their perceived lack of moral and sexual restraint became an accepted cause of immorality. Signs of independence by older women attracted reprobation, at least until the later eighteenth century when women were recast in a passive role and the menopause, until then a very natural phenomenon, was brought firmly into the realm of the burgeoning medical profession. Those who subdue you first have to crush or humiliate you.

Many of these early modern physicians assumed that 'modest-minded women' were keeping their ailments to themselves through a rightful feminine shame. The first English gynaecological handbook had been written by a woman for other women because they were 'ashamed to reveal and tell their distress to any man'. They were also at risk of being very badly received by men aware of their complaints:

> although women have various maladies and more terrible sicknesses than any man knows, as I said, they are ashamed for fear of reproof in times to come and of disclosure by discourteous men who love women only for physical pleasure and for evil gratification. And if women are sick, such men despise them and fail to realize how much sickness women have before they bring them into this world. And so, to assist women, I intend to write of how to help their secret maladies so that one woman may aid another in her illness and not divulge her secrets to such discourteous men; for he despises not only women but God who sends such sickness in their best interests.[45]

In the seventeenth century a 'Doctor in Physicke at Norwich', John Sadler, published *The Sicke Womans Private Looking-Glasse*

(1636) to give women the words 'to informe the Physician about the cause of their griefe' and thereby avoid the affront their bodies afforded them. Having consulted his Galenic and Hippocratic texts, he concluded that

> amongst all diseases incident to the body, I found none more frequent, none more perilous than those which arise from the ill-affected wombe: for through the evill quality thereof, the heart, the liver, and the braine are affected; from whence the actions vitall, natural, & animal are hurt.

Women, through their 'ignorance and modestie', were subject to 'manifold distempers of body' and, he said, were apparently 'so shamefac'd and modest' that they would rather suffer all their discomforts than reveal themselves by consulting a physician.[46] Knowledge of the body was power and medical writers attempted to keep control of the information by writing much of it in Latin, thereby limiting it to the educated only, for which read 'men'.[47] A few medical texts were written in plain English so that women who wished to might treat themselves, and authors tried to assure women at the outset that the works would not outrage feminine modesty; either that or they were sensibly trying to deflect any criticism of their chosen subject. An attack on physicians in 1670 spoke of 'Groaping Doctors' who pretended they could not treat a woman without touching her, something that was thought undignified at best. Physical examinations were rarely carried out until the beginning of the nineteenth century, though most women consulted not physicians or apothecaries but midwives and, of course, they discussed their ills amongst themselves. The ignorance or fraudulence of a physician, however, was rarely commented upon.

Equality of male and female medical practitioners was unheard of until fairly recently, and there were no hard and fast rules as to what constituted a female 'medical practitioner'. They were usually referred to as midwives (an amorphous group with no institutional identity, no guilds, and not formally licensed before the early to mid fifteenth century), nurses and *vetulae*. The latter, a very common term, actually means nothing more than 'old woman' but, through the disparagement cultivated by physicians and learned surgeons attempting to denigrate their competitors in the medical marketplace, *vetulae* came to stand for all that was ignorant, illiterate, rustic and superstitious. They were lumped together with other despised groups such as 'barbers, fortune-tellers, *locatores*, *insidiatores*, tricksters, alchemists, prostitutes, midwives, converted Jews, and Muslims'. Informal medical practice was widespread enough among women to worry the male physicians and surgeons, and although there were regulations being put in place to restrict the medical work of women they could never be universally enforced.[48]

Jakob Sprenger and Heinrick Kramer, Dominican monks and authors of the *Malleus Maleficarum* (*The Hammer of Witches*), first published in 1486, used the rhetoric of witchcraft not so much against midwives as against the *vetulae* and empirics, though the timing of midwifery regulations coincided with the first stirrings of the early modern wave of witch persecutions. Petitions had been put to Parliament in the fourteenth century about the 'worthless and presumptuous women' who usurped the medical profession, and asked for fines and imprisonment of women who tried to 'use the practise of Fisyk'. The Church proclaimed that 'if a woman dare to cure *without having studied* she is a witch and must die,' though there was no way for a woman to go to university or study medicine. The 'greatest injuries to the Faith as regards the heresy of witches are done by midwives', said the Inquisitors, 'and this is made clearer than daylight itself by the confessions of some who were afterwards burned'.[49] In England in 1511 an Act was passed by which physicians tried to limit the practice of empirics and roundly condemned 'women [who] boldly and accustomably take upon them great Cures, and things of great difficulty, in which they partly use Sorcery or Witchcraft'.[50] A hundred years later, in 1619, Samuel Purchas berated women who chose other women to treat their illnesses, asking, 'How many old Women preferred before their greatest Doctor?', though the best and most expensive physicians and surgeons were no guarantee of health.[51] At the same time as older women were becoming patients they were being squeezed out of the healing role.

A meeting of the College of Physicians of London in 1583 discussed the threat to their status by the older women practising medicine. They would have to control them whilst battling against the prevailing idea that the women knew more and caused less harm than they did. Less visible than the educated gentlemen, these women were everywhere, and were labelled by them as poor, ignorant, bold, blind, stubborn and demented. If they lived without men they were considered a major part of the burden of dependency, measured by the compulsory poor rate from the sixteenth century, and they became subject to the late-sixteenth- and seventeenth-century 'crisis of misogyny'. Barely registering on the male medical radar, they could evade censure only by working quietly in the prescribed 'women's realm'.

The older woman's perceived power and sexuality were manifest in the idea of witches – the thousands of older women who might turn the natural, social and divine orders upside down – and redolent in the terrifying fear that they might seek demonic lovers to satisfy their extreme lusts. Such voraciousness was suspected particularly when the woman was widowed or single with no legitimate sexual outlet and at her most vulnerable to devilish seduction. Such women were allegedly sealing their pacts with the Devil by performing all manner of sexual acts with him, kissing his buttocks as well as causing impotence, barrenness, miscarriage and infant death.[52] 'Every night,' writes the historian Hugh Trevor-Roper, 'these ill-advised ladies were anointing themselves with the "devil's grease", made out of the fat of murdered infants, and, thus lubricated, were slipping through cracks and keyholes and up chimneys, mounting on broomsticks or spindles or airborne goats, and flying off on a long and inexpressibly wearisome journey to a diabolical rendezvous, the witch's sabat.'[53] They indulged in parodies of the Eucharist and went from being practitioners of simple harmful deeds, *maleficia*, to being a mass, heretical, rebellious and, most importantly, diabolical movement, a threat to the Christian society. Augustine's arguments against magic, differentiating it from miracle, were a crucial element in the denunciation of witches and their sacrilegious craft by the early Church. 'Thou shalt not suffer a witch to live,' it is declared in Exodus 22:18 in the King James VI Bible.[54] A misogynist Church claimed the Latin word '*femina*' (woman) was from the Spanish word '*fe*' (faith) and the Latin word '*mina*' (less) as, since the fall of Eve, women were apparently less able to resist their appetites and the Devil's marvellously seductive ways.[55]

These women might experience uncontrollable sexual wants, 'insane love', the precursor of *furor uterinus* or nymphomania. Cases appeared in Britain and across Europe during the sixteenth and seventeenth centuries. Girolamo, a sixteenth-century Italian physician, defined it as 'an immoderate burning in the genital area of the female, caused by the surging of hot vapour, bringing about an erection of the clitoris',[56] and this burning sensation was thought to drive women quite mad. In the seventeenth century, Felix Platter described a matron 'who was in every other way most honourable, but who invited by the basest words and gestures men and dogs to have intercourse with her'. She was, he thought, possessed by the Devil, whose 'diseases and remedies exceed the limits and boundaries of Nature'.[57]

At early witchcraft trials in Europe both men and women were put to death, though it was not long before women represented the majority of victims. An average of 80 per cent were female and the majority of these were older. Often marginal, weak and unpopular, about 64 per cent were widowed and half of these lived alone (at the beginning of the seventeenth century 3.5–7.5 per cent of all women were widowed, a figure which increased to 10–20 per cent in years of war). Young women eventually became targets too: in Germany in 1582, since they had 'all but eradicated the old ones, we will now go after the young'.[58] Being menopausal, and hence a sick and irrational creature, was occasionally used as a defence in law, thus colluding in and strengthening a destructive female stereotype. The notion of unruly women as scapegoats for social evils and the accompanying misogynistic rhetoric is nothing new and neither is the willingness or need of women in some cultures to exploit it.[59]

Continental ideas about the nature and practices of witchcraft gradually seeped into Britain from Europe through learned treatises such as the *Malleus Maleficarum* and the *Guide to Grand Iury Men* (1627), and all sorts and ranks of society played a significant role in the prosecution of witches, believing that they were a threat to the status quo.[60]

Over half of the women arraigned for witchcraft in 1645 in Essex, England, were unmarried or widows. It seems that those prosecuted for witchcraft were on the whole poor compared with their alleged victims, and that resentment and envy were causes of social tension, often based on a neighbour denying economic assistance.[61] Contemporary commentators noted that the most common emotion demonstrated by accused witches was discontent and a desire for revenge, perhaps unsurprisingly, given how nightmarish their circumstances could be. The numbers of poor and needy must have seemed overwhelming in the seventeenth century after a series of disastrous harvests. More people were reliant on poor relief, especially the lone, elderly female, traditionally an economic drain on parish resources. A clergyman, John Gaul, exasperated with the wild anxieties of the people, wrote in his *Selected Cases of Conscience touching Witches and Witchcraft* (1646) that

> Every old woman with a wrinkled face, a furred brow, a hairy lip, a gobber tooth, a squint eye, a squeaking voice, or a scolding tongue, having a rugged coat on her back, a skull cap on her head, a spindle in her hand, and a dog or cat by her side, is not only suspected, but pronounced for a witch.

The last execution of witches in England took place in 1684, in France in 1745, Germany 1775, Switzerland 1782 and in Poland in 1792, but some people continued to believe in witches long after.[62] Samuel Taylor Coleridge, travelling in Germany at the very end of the eighteenth century, recorded the insignia against witchcraft that he saw:

both on Inns, Stables, & Farms there are ALWAYS nailed up at both Gables two pieces of wood . . . the crosses often shaped into horns & horses heads. This, they believe universally, keeps off the Evil Spirit who in a ball of fire would come into their chimneys. – Here *all* the higher classes, except the Clergy *perhaps*, are Infidels – all the *People* grossly superstitious.

In America the executions ended after the Salem witch panic that infested Essex County, Massachusetts, in 1692.[63] The accused were overwhelmingly women. Puritans, many of whom were dissenters driven away from East Anglia by religious persecution, did not believe that the women amongst them were by nature more evil than men, but they did 'know' them to be weaker and more susceptible to sinful impulses. Post-menopausal women were particularly vulnerable as they no longer served the purpose of procreation. If widowed, they neither fulfilled the role of wife nor were they protected by a husband from malicious accusations, and women who inherited property violated the common expectations that wealth should pass down the male line. Their precarious situation led them into conflict with others and any aggressive or contentious behaviour on their part might bring them grave troubles. The widows Bridget Bishop and Susannah Martin were both executed in 1692. Bishop had inherited her first husband's property before remarrying and Martin had attempted, unsuccessfully, to secure through litigation her father's estate, which she believed to be her rightful inheritance. Many of the accused were known for their healing skills, occult expertise and divination. Benign or otherwise, they were then open to suspicion and attack. Puritans believed in a close connection between heresy, heathenism and witchcraft, and a significant number of the accused had Quaker associations. Some were linked by their accusers to Native Americans. Tituba, a Native American woman who had lived in the Caribbean before coming with her master to Salem, was attacked because of her 'difference' as well as her reputation for occult skills. By the time the trials were halted in October 1692 nineteen people had been hanged, thirteen of whom were women. In addition to the Salem trials another sixty-one proceedings are known to have taken place in New England during the seventeenth century.[64]

The spread of witch trials in the years of the Renaissance and the Reformation reflected fierce tensions in society as older systems of belief broke down.[65] Wise or cunning women who held arcane knowledge on the use and properties of plants and knew how to control their own fertility were feared because they might not submit to the prevailing educated male elite. The witch, often the female physician of the Middle Ages, was an obstacle to male dominance and the development of modern medicine.[66] Her skills would be denigrated and her mind and body would be appropriated and subdued by other means than burning.

The menopause was mentioned only in oblique fashion in medical writing before the seventeenth century. There was no specific term for it and little attention was paid to it compared with abundant discussion of how to stimulate and maintain menstruation. The list of symptoms of this 'enfer des femmes', this women's hell, however, was growing in length and miserable detail. Almost every possible disorder or disease was now linked to the menopause. Women might experience sensations of pain in the loins and legs, loss of appetite, deafness, migraines, dizziness and sudden flushes of the face followed by sweatings and chills, dizziness and fainting, vomiting, nausea, increased urinary, bronchial and lacrimary secretion, frequent yawning, hiccups, palpitations, greater sensitivity, agitation, indifference to pleasure, sadness, 'upset against her children, her husband, those around her', violent outbursts, strange fears and sensations. Individual crasis, or temperament, and a woman's environment were also believed to influence her experiences: thin women were thought to absorb the excess blood into fat; too much blood still would be lost through nosebleeds, haemorrhoids, coughing or vomiting as a form of substitute menstruation. The prevailing orthodox medical knowledge maintained that the menopause was a consequence of ageing whereby the blood and fibres thickened and hardened with time and gave rise to a list of foul and ghastly consequences.[67]

There appeared to be no escape from this miserable end, and to compound her physical decline a woman might also have to endure the contempt of a society which could not allow her to 'flout nature'. Post-menopausal women, redundant members of 'that viler Sex', according to John Oldham (1653–83), were nothing but lost and 'nasty' souls. With barbaric wishful thinking he argued that, were they trees 'without fruit', they would 'be hewn down and cast into the fire'.[68] Love and all chance of it should be a thing of their past, he railed. Sexual love was not for older women, who flouted nature with their desires and attempts to attract lovers. Richard Braithwait, in *The English Gentleman; and the English Gentlewoman* (1641), agreed:

When maids are deepe struck in years, be their fortunes never so promising, their alliance strengthening, or the beauty of their inward parts deserving; they are commonly courted by youthfull fancy, with a neglect full of contempt. Their rivell'd skin merits not a light amorous touch; nor their rugged browes deepe-indented with aged furrows, a gracefull looke.[69]

The scornful Robert Gould saw nothing but 'pale rottenness, and ashes' in those who practised surface deceit with 'curled Locks', 'Glas eye', 'Ivory Tooth' and 'artificial Buttocks'. Swift's cruelly satiric poem aimed at older women, 'A Beautiful Young Nymph Going to Bed' (1731), tells of one Corinna's bedtime routine:

> Now, picking out a crystal eye,
> She wipes it clean, and lays it by.
> Her eyebrows from a mouse's hide,
> Stuck on with art on either side,
> Pulls off with care, and first displays 'em,
> Then in a play-book smoothly lays 'em.
> Now dextrously her plumpers draws,
> That serve to fill her hollow jaws.
> Untwists a wire; and from her gums
> A set of teeth completely comes.
> Pulls out the rags contriv'd to prop
> Her flabby dugs, and down they drop . . .
>
> The nymph, though in this mangled plight,
> Must every morn her limbs unite.
> But how shall I describe her arts
> To recollect the scattered parts?
> Or show the anguish, toil, and pain,
> Of gathering up herself again?

Not only did the menopause signal a loss of desirability, it meant that women should severely curb their behaviour and preferably keep quiet, even disappear altogether. Thomas Becon's *A new catechism* (1564) advised silence, but if she did open her mouth she should

> so speak as it becometh women of gravitie . . . without reproach or ignominies to other. . . . nothing doth so greatly provoke olde women into babbling, as too much drinking (for when the wine is in, the wit is out) and old women naturally love well-tippling: the holy Apostle [St Paul] commandeth that the ancient matrons shall not give themselves too much wine but rather embrace sobriety and temperancy . . . drunkenness is the mother and nurse of many lewd vices in old women, which ought to be Mistresses of sobriety and mirrors of all virtue, it is not only vile and in-commendable, but horrible and detestable. For an old woman overcome with drunkenness, is made a sink of all evils.

Women were a little less cruel to their sisters but still warned of what could be expected in old age. Hannah Woolley, in her handbook *The Gentlewoman's Companion or, a Guide to the Female Sex: containing Directions of Behaviour, in all Places, Companies, Relations, and Conditions, from their Childhood down to Old Age* (London, 1675), bemoaned the unfairness of it:

> alas, what would become of a great many to whom Nature hath proved an unkind Stepmother, denying them not only convenient use of members, but hath thrown on them deformity of parts; these corporal incommodities would make them pass for monsters, did not the excellency of their Souls compensate these irreparable defects.

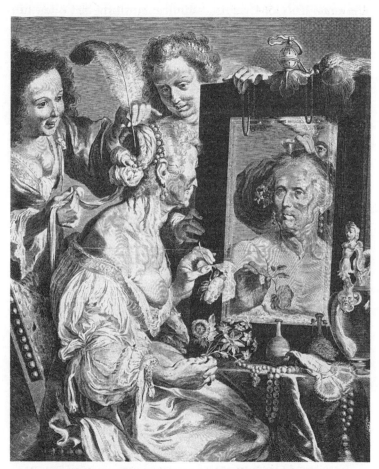

A cruel stab at the 'vanity' of old age when beauty, youth and fecundity were the be all and end all of women.

If Nature hath deni'd me what is fit,
The Want of Beauty I repay with Wit!

The first 'Rule of Civility, which is nothing but a certain
Modesty or *Pudor*' is 'Ladies, you must consult your years,
and so accordingly behave your self to your age and condition. Next, preserve all due respect to the quality of the
Person you converse withal. Thirdly consider well the
Time. And, lastly, the place where you are . . . For an old
woman to habit her self as youthfully as a gentlewoman of
fifteen, is as improper as to sing a wanton song at a
Funeral.'

Domestic remedy books written by women had flourished in the sixteenth and seventeenth centuries before
the disenfranchisement of the female lay-healers and the
increasing monopoly of medical care by professionally
regulated male physicians calling on the authority of new
'science'. These diverse and eclectic books were extremely
important when good health was a fickle thing and were
handed down from mother to daughter, a continuous and
dynamic record of everyday domestic living. The medical
recipes they held were often promiscuously mixed with
cookery and cosmetic recipes, their ingredients and methods of preparation frequently overlapping and covering
all manner of administrations with waters, ointments,
puddings, potions, poultices and purgatives. As in life, the
serious sat side by side with the frivolous: Dorcas Gwynne's
mid-seventeenth-century book at one point runs, 'to make
a custard; to make a hedghogg pudding; a medicine for all
manner of bruises' and an 'almond milk against abound-
ance of heate whereby the head or body is distempered'.[70]
Hannah Woolley's book included a recipe to 'preserve her

face and reduce her flushes' and recommended that 'to cleanse the skin of the face, and it look beautiful and fair . . . take Rosemary and boil it in White-wine, with the juice of Erigan put thereunto, and wash your face therewith Mornings and Evenings. If your face be troubled with heat, take Elder-flowers, Plantane, white Daisie-roots, and Herb-Robert and put these into running-water, and wash your Face therewith at night, and in the Morning'.[71]

George Saville's *The Lady's New Year's Gift, Or, Advice to a Daughter* (1707) gave advice on religion, husbands, house-hold matters, family and children, behaviour and conver-sation, friendships, censure, vanity and affectation, pride, diversions, and he added 'one *Advice* to conclude . . . which is that you let every seven years make some alteration in you towards the *Graver* side, and not be like the *Girls* of Fifty, who *resolve* to be always *Young*, whatever *Time* with his Iron Teeth hath determined to the contrary'. Such mockery for the '*Girls* of Fifty' bubbled over into hostile mirth at their expense, and male jokes about the female body and its perceived absurdities descended into outright aggression designed to humiliate and reduce.[72] Benjamin Franklin's essay 'Advice to a young man on the choice of a mistress' (1745) easily proffered more than one such satirical reason, for example, why an inexperienced male youth might seek out an older woman. Her charms being compromised by the years, he thought it most conven-ient that she aged from the top down, allowing her lower parts to be 'as much enjoyed as if she were young'.[73] Enlarging on his subject, Franklin instructed the young man that

The face first grows lank and wrinkled; then the neck; then
the breast and arms; the lower parts continuing to the
last as plump as ever: so that covering all above with a basket,
and regarding only what is below the girdle, it is impossible of two women to know an old from a young one. And
as in the dark all cats are grey, the pleasure of corporeal
enjoyment with an old woman is at least equal, and frequently superior, every knack being by practice capable of
improvement.

It could be that eighteenth-century men and women did not
recognize this condescending and parodic impulse as misogynistic, the term having been recorded first in 1656 to signify
hatred of or contempt for women. Recognized or not, the
vile negative assumptions about older women as inherently
pathological, pointless or just plain unpleasant were invidi-
ous and ingrained.

For 1500 years, such views had dominated. Medical knowledge was still based on classical medical and philosophical
texts; Aristotle and Galen remained the supreme authorities
in the sciences and biology. Most scholars were versed in
mathematics, botany, chemistry, optics, philosophy, mysti-
cism, anatomy, experimental physiology and from the
seventeenth century they began to branch off and specialize
in particular areas of medicine. Gynaecology was one. The
drive to differentiate between orthodox and unorthodox
healers, to make distinct the division between traditional
medieval ways and modern scientific medicine, now became
paramount. The menopause had barely existed on any
medical radar before the eighteenth century let alone made
grand appearances in the nosologies and other works on
pathology. Where it was written about it was portrayed as a

natural and expected occurrence, albeit with very negative overtones. Women had simply got on with it amongst themselves for centuries but orthodox medicine was about to make itself indispensable to menopausal women.

3

THEIR NATURE EXPLAINED

'Autrefois quand j'étais femme' (Once, when I was a woman)

Madame de Deffand, quoted in Tilt, E. J.,
The Change of Life in Health and Disease

In the relentless rise of science, anatomists began to define a woman's fertility with their knives, and physicians began to refine their knowledge of her functions. The deeper examination of the female body began and ended, as always, with reproduction. Fertility determined a woman's being; the end of fertility nullified her. The menopause was a mere afterthought, a footnote, an end of interest and a precursor of trouble.

In 1555 the celebrated anatomist Versalius had described the ovaries as the 'female testicles'; a hundred years later Stensen pointed out that, as they contained ova, they should be called ovaries. Fallopius, an anatomist of Modena and Venice, pupil of Versalius, described the corpus luteum in 1561, overturning the assumption that the ovaries contained semen. He described the tubes named after him thus: 'That slender and narrow seminal passage rises from the horn of the uterus very white and sinewy but after it has passed outward a little way it becomes gradually broader and curls like the tendrils of a vine.'[1] It would be another 200 years before surgeons, noting that women who had had their ovaries removed ceased to menstruate, would conclude in an opaque manner that menstruation was due to a 'peculiar condition of the ovaries'.

The process of ovulation and the Graafian follicles were described by the young physician Reinier de Graaf in 1672. He was in his twenties when he worked on his influential essay, 'New treatise concerning the generative organs of women', published in Latin the year before he died but not translated into English until 300 years later. In *On the organs of women which serve the purpose of procreation* (Leiden, 1672) he gave a detailed account of ovaries and their essential importance, unrecognized from Aristotle to William Harvey. With biblical authority and a touch of serious playfulness, he wrote, after Proverbs chapter 30, 'there are three things which are insatiable: . . . hell, and the os vulvae, and earth'.[2]

De Graaf's work was more detailed and revelatory than any previous publication on the subject and he is considered by some to be the 'first modern reproductive biologist'. His brief life was intense and intensely productive; fascinated by his subject, he recorded his knowledge and ideas with meticulous words and beautiful, credible, anatomical drawings. Born in the Netherlands, brought up a Roman Catholic in a predominantly Calvinist country, he studied medicine in Germany and France, eventually settling in Delft in 1666 where he began his influential work. But he died very young, probably of the plague, just one year after his marriage, aged thirty-two.[3]

De Graaf was, like the rest of his profession, concerned about possible accusations of salacious activity and at pains to say that he 'described the genital parts, not to encourage seduction, and indulgence in pleasure but to improve men's knowledge of themselves for the benefit of the medical community'. To this end, he was the first to elaborate on the clitoris in detail. Whereas, previously, it had been understood as a small penis, a nugatory quasi-male appendage, he emphasized its difference and its abundant innervation and function. 'The glans of the clitoris,' he wrote,

> is endowed with such sharpened perceptive sensitivity that it is not without justice called the sweetness of love, the gad-fly of Venus. Indeed, if these parts of the pudendum had not been endowed with such an exquisite sensitivity to pleasure and passion, no woman would be willing to take upon herself the irksome nine-months-long business of gestation, the painful and often fatal process of expelling the fetus and the worrisome and care-ridden task of raising children.[4]

The function of women's sexual pleasure fascinated him. The paraurethral glands, which he termed the 'female prostate', existed to

> generate a serous juice which makes women more libidinous and lubricates their sexual parts in agreeable fashion during coitus. Here too it should be noted that the discharge from the female 'prostate' causes as much pleasure as does that from the male . . . I mean those females who, with lascivious thoughts, frisky fingers or instruments devised contrary to decent morals, wickedly stir themselves up to such a pitch that they eject copious quantities of this kind of matter.

De Graaf has been credited with discovering the G-spot (first described 200 years later by Gräfenberg) and he believed that the function of the vagina is 'simply to constrict, where necessary, the part it embraces, particularly at the time of coitus', and found it so cleverly constructed that it would accommodate itself to 'each and every penis; it will grow out to meet a short one, retire before a long one, dilate for a fat one, and constrict for a thin one'. Reassuring his fellows that nature had 'taken account of every variety of penis', de Graaf informed them that there was no need to seek a 'scabbard the same size as your knife', for women, fascinating as they might be, were designed for the convenience of men.

His treatise contains chapters on the clitoris, hymen, menstrual flow, ovaries and the existence of 'albumen in women's eggs' which could be 'quite prettily demonstrated by boiling them'. The liquid in the eggs 'acquires from being boiled the same colour, flavour and consistency as does the albumen in fowl's eggs'. De Graaf had to use the same methods as many of his peers to make his discoveries, that is, an empirical, hands-on experiment, which in this case meant cooking and eating the eggs from a cadaver. But, despite the scope of his work, de Graaf's interest in the ovaries stopped when their reproductive use was no longer viable. His work contains no chapter on, no mention even of, the cessation of the menses, yet his revolutionary approach to women and their experience of reproduction did introduce a new way of looking at female health. He described women's experiences of pregnancy, childbirth and menstruation, and he considered the bodily sensations women derived from such experiences. This was foreign territory to the majority of the male medical profession.

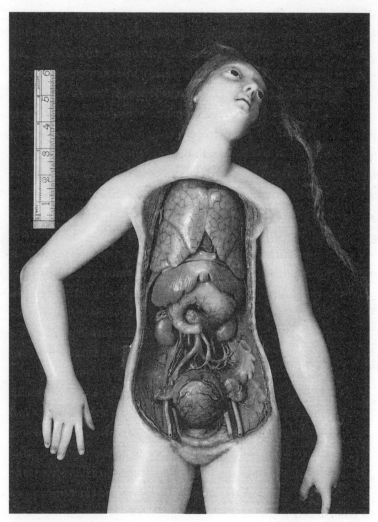

A chillingly realistic, eighteenth-century wax figure revealing the female anatomy.

The modern menopause as disease really began here and the first known monograph on the subject was published in 1710 by Simon David Titius. It concentrated, unsurprisingly, on the negative, 'treatable' aspects of the menopause. Similar works followed and soon the menopause joined the worst of all the 'calamities' to beset 'a sex that seems destined to support the largest share of human misery'.[5] They set the scene for future fear, dread, trouble and misery. The new works merely continued the prejudices and peculiarities of previous ideas but anecdotal and fearsome myths were now couched in a more modern, 'scientific' language by orthodox physicians, bestowing credibility upon them. Treatments and assumptions initially barely changed.

Physicians tried to reassure women that they were going through a natural physiological process, but their intervention was necessarily disease-orientated and what was altruistic also became a constraint. An anonymous physician wrote in 1739 that

> it will not be amiss to touch upon the Disorders that most Women labour under, when being between forty and fifty years of Age, their *Courses* begin first to dodge and at last to leave them; for then they are frequently troubled with a Severe Pain in the Head and Back, and about the Loins; oftimes also with Cholick Pains, Gripes, and Looseness, at other Times with Vapours to a Violent Degree; likewise feverish Heats, wandering Rheumatick Pains and general Uneasiness.

He recommended phlebotomy, removing 8 ozs of blood and 'After [this] no Method, or Medicine, are more proper or beneficial than my *Purging Pills*' in tandem with 'my Uterine

Drops'. These preparations he advertised for sale at 3s 6d an item, a very expensive treatment regime in the early eighteenth century. The use of emmenagogues to alleviate stagnating blood, such as leeches to the genitalia and the cervix, and the encouragement of vicarious menstruation via haemorrhoids, nosebleeds and phlebotomies (but only in the waxing of the moon) were the first port of call in treating the cessation of bleeding. Purgation and excretion through the skin remained popular, too, by vesicatories, cupping, issues, cauteries, setons, sweating and bathing. These procedures sometimes caused iatrogenic (physician-induced) ills: the backache and pains in the loins described could equally have been caused by the emmenagogues affecting the urinary tract and causing strangury, cholick, gripes and looseness. The French novelist and playwright Alain-René Lesage (1668–1747), in his classic novel *Gil Blas* (1715), describes a lively woman of indeterminate age who kept her youth through two open issues – one on each buttock. Such familiarity with bleeding didn't come naturally according to the influential Scottish obstetrician William Smellie, who suggested that young girls were often frightened witless at their first period. Describing the rush of blood, he recounted how they became so '*distended* with [it] that their sphincters or mouths [were] forced *open*'. It was said of Smellie that no one could discuss the subject of midwifery without referring to his detailed and accurate book, but he had his critics: the midwife Elizabeth Nihell, in defence of female knowledge in the profession of midwifery, said, with some feeling, that he had the 'delicate fist of a great-horse-godmother of a he-midwife'.[6] John Anderson, in his *Medical Remarks on Natural, Spontaneous and Artificial Evacuation* (London, 1787), offered two fatal cases of what he considered to be spontaneous vicarious menstrual bleeding when the catamenia have 'ceased to flow by the vagina' and made 'choice of some other emunctory' such as 'that of the mouth'. If bleeding happened to return after the usual final period, as it sometimes did, he thought it 'occasioned by some exciting cause; which if not removed will be fatal'. It was of the utmost consequence to restore menstruation and, adhering to ancient ideas about the suppression of bleeding and stagnating blood, he believed it would 'acquire new qualities, habitudes, positions, detominations and relations', and 'mania is not an uncommon effect'.[7]

In his *Emmenologia*, Freind castigated his over-enthusiastic peers who had been 'led away by their fancies' and 'proved rather Interpreters of their own Dreams than of Nature'. Here was a man of literature, medicine and natural philosophy, involved in some of the major political events of his time: he wrote his influential work *A History of Physick from the Time of Galen to the beginning of the Sixteenth Century* (1725–6) whilst imprisoned in the Tower for his Jacobite activities. There is 'hardly any Argument, on which Physicians have wrote more', he said, mainly because they understood it so little, but 'almost all the Distempers, with which the women are afflicted, are derived, as Hippocrates well observed, from some irregularity of the Menses'. 'Wretched surely and unequal,' he continued,

> seems the condition of the Female Sex, that they who are by Nature destined to be the Preservers of the human Race, should at the same time be made liable to so many Diseases. For whatever Course of Life they pursue, few there are, who enjoy an Health untainted and exempt from Pain: for if they enter into a wedded State, even from that Source of Pleasures

something bitter arises, and Pregnancy brings with it at least
a length of loathing, if nothing more calamitous; if they
make a Vow of Celibacy, with all their precaution they will
hardly be able to avoid labouring under some Distemper,
even upon that very account, because they are strangers to a
Mothers pangs.

Paradoxically, he seemed to suggest that all these terrible
trials would 'cease at the *seventh Septenary* without an injury to
Health' as women become 'destitute of the Menses'.[8]

Definitions of menstruation were very fluid at this time
and any periodic discharge of blood might be referred to as
such, even if it was a man experiencing it in the form of
haemorrhoids or haemorrhages. By 1800, however, most
medical theorists had concluded that menstruation was limited to the female sex and flowed from the uterus or vagina
alone, establishing a significant sex difference.[9] Physicians
began to take greater interest in their 'new' patients, to discover more about them, and the male medical profession
encroached more forcefully and speedily on the role of the
female midwife in pursuit of work, money, status and knowledge.[10] This doesn't mean that ancient beliefs were sloughed
off. Rather, they were embraced. It was a process of absorp-
tion and embellishment. According to medical opinion there
were powerful physical and moral reasons for a woman's
social subordination and, since the menstrual cycle was
linked to the phases of the moon and the female body was
constantly in flux, she was both physiologically and psychologically unstable, in need of control and constitutionally
prone to madness. The continual state of female ill-health
needed regulation in ways that male health did not. The
Galenic idea of women's limited and domestic role being

determined by nature rather than culture was reinforced. Women in warmer climes, for example, were considered to menstruate more freely and frequently, so their northern sisters were encouraged to keep warm by cooking in the kitchens, doing laundry and having lots of sex.[11] Women's sedentary domestic lives were organized by nature and nature would provide the remedies as the physicians could not; they could act only as knowledgeable mediators.

The workings of women's bodies, their very nature, were known to be a distortion. When Martin Schurig of Dresden published *Gynaecologia* in 1730, a work on the diseases peculiar to women, it also covered perceived deviations such as fornication, rape, vaginismus, nymphomania, chastity, lesbianism, buggery and bestiality.[12] Astruc's *A Treatise on all the Diseases Incident to Women* (1740) supported the subjective role of women and the dire effects of their natural excessive lewdness. Affirming that women and other female animals bled, 'particularly *Bitches* when proud', he thought women akin to beasts. Many agreed that 'no animal is subject to *Catamenia* but Women and Apes'. Astruc was a French Royal Physician and Regis Professor in Paris when his work was translated from a manuscript copy of his lectures in 1740. In his treatise Astruc reveals the lack of understanding and trust, not to mention the necessary deceit that could prevail between a male physician and a female patient: 'If the patient be a widow or unmarried, though she be with child, she will rarely tell the Truth.' John Leake, a man-midwife writing in 1777, thought that women's nature was riddled with 'erring reason' and they were subject to 'the tyranny and prevalence of pernicious customs'.

Despite his prejudices Leake was a compassionate man: he was a member of the Royal College of Physicians and

founder of the Westminster Lying-in Hospital, a charity
which most unusually admitted single women (though they
were allowed one chance only).[13] Both Astruc and Leake
dismissed the ancient belief in menstrual blood as 'ranked
among Poysons; that they withered and dried up the
Flowers, marr'd Liquors [and] tarnished Looking-Glasses'.
Astruc noted that this secretion was 'as good and balsamic as
any' and merely a 'nutritious Juice redundant in the Body'.
It could not be 'malignant', asserted Leake, because it was the
same fluid used to nourish a child in the womb, and this
'critical evacuation' was not to 'purify blood from something malignant or poisonous; but only . . . an expedient to
prevent a *Plethora*, or overfulness of the vessels'. If, however,
the blood had 'stagnated too long in the womb' it still might
'acquire pernicious qualities and, taken back into circulation, could be dangerous, unwholesome, corrupt, depraved
by being too long at rest'. Even a woman's blood shouldn't
rest.

The 'Cessation of the Periodical Discharge in the Decline
of Life', according to Leake, was 'the very reverse' of what
happens at menarche: the 'long accustomed evacuation will
entirely cease; and with it the faculty of having children' —
the 'tide of nature being turned'. With 'declining Menstrua'
the '*uterine Vessels* [once] flexible and open, become rigid and
contracted' and the 'Quantity [of Chyle] may become less
than usual; the Quality may be changed . . . the Duration
may be shorter . . . the Menstrua may appear but once in
two or three months'. The vessels 'gradually become
corrupted, dry and hard, just as by age it happens to the
visible Parts of the Body, particularly the Skin of the Face,
and above all, the Substance of the Breasts'. The blood col-
lects, Astruc says, and women begin to suffer headaches,

haemorrhages, weakness, convulsive and 'hysterick Motions, Pains of the Loins, Fits, intense Redness of the Face, Regurgitation of *uterine Milk* into the Blood, difficulty with Respiration, pains of the *Matrix*, *Pica*, and *Malacia*' and 'all the Symptoms which attended before . . . appear now without any Flux'. The symptoms, he writes, commonly 'decrease gradually . . . and [it] rarely demands the Attendance of the Physician'.[14]

Not so, according to Henry Manning, who roundly damned Astruc in 1771 as a superfluous, whimsical man with 'arbitrary, theoretical opinions'. It was not in the least helpful, he ranted, that physicians such as Astruc, with their 'many absurd endeavours [and] a thousand idle and ridiculous notions' had caused the subject of the menses, 'obscure in its own nature', to be 'rendered still more intricate'. Manning understood quite clearly, through his observations, that 'the diseases of that sex depend principally on the excess or diminution of the menstrual discharge', no more, no less. In healthy women menstruation proceeds 'in an uniform course to the years of forty or forty-five; at which time the periods become gradually more irregular and protracted to the decline of life, which, in this temperate climate, is commonly estimated at the age of fifty'. However, there are many instances that he records of bleeding continuing to an advanced age and even pregnancies in later years, though these might prove to be 'False Conceptions and Moles . . . a shapeless mass of matter, partly of a membraneous and partly of a fleshy appearance, of which women are sometimes delivered, with pains and other symptoms resembling those of real labour'. The false pregnancies were 'owing chiefly to coagulated blood . . . There have been instances of women who have gone with moles for several years' and they were most common

with those who are in the decline of life, on account of the
great obstructions to which such women are liable, from the
irregularity of their periods; in consequence of which, the
retained blood being strongly pressed by the action of the
uterus, its ferrous parts are forced off, and the fibrous portion
is compacted into a firm substance of a fleshy appearance.

This critical period of life is usually attended, he said, with a
variety of complaints, the most common of which are 'ver-
tigo, headache, rheumatic pains, hysteric affections, fevers
and inflammations of different kinds, bloody urine, and
unusual hemorrhages from the lungs, nose, and other
parts . . . these are either prevented, or relieved, by a reasonable use of the lancet, and other evacuations, a cooling diet,
and temperate regime'.[15]

Although physicians were keen to emphasize the differences
between the sexes, to bring order and diagnose, and whilst
they risked parodying the 'fair sex', they also sympathized.
Chauvinistic and patronizing as it may seem today there
was a strong element of altruism in the medical profession.
Physicians wanted to improve women's lot, cursed as they
seemed to be with 'unruly' bodies enervated by the demands
of their reproductive task. Women, too, were not above using
what power they had at their disposal by exploiting their alleged
sensibilities and acting over-excited, exhausted and without
self-control.[16] The construct of the weak and childish woman,
even if it could sometimes be turned to useful effect, was never
going to be a good thing in the long run, though that doesn't
seem to have diminished its popularity.

Flighty feebleness of intellect and a love of excess seemed to
afflict most women, according to the majority of eighteenth-
century medical texts. Leake's work was 'principally intended

for the *Female Sex*', who, he said, 'often regard unimportant knowledge, whilst they neglect the means of being sufficiently acquainted with what concerns their health'. He avoids detailed discussion of the female body because this 'would rather embarrass and perplex than instruct' women, who are far more interested in the 'extremes of fashion and false ornament', so he beguiles them by saying that 'altho' health does not altogether constitute beauty; beauty is the child of health, and cannot exist long without her parental influence'. Leake knew that women coveted beauty, though he didn't acknowledge that their lives or livelihood might have depended upon it; rather he castigated them for vanity whilst playing on it so as to 'teach [them] to trust *Regimen* and *Simple Medicines*'. All 'Weakness and inward Decay' would be banished and beauty be theirs if they followed his instruction, for it was health 'which animates and lights up the countenance with expressive and bewitching smiles; which touches the lips with vermillion, and diffuses o'er the cheeks a freshness and vivid glow surpassing circassian bloom; it gives balmy sweetness to the breath, and lustre to the eye'. Still, he grumbled, 'the idea of every woman being her own physician is ludicrous' as she holds so 'many peculiar errors and absurd opinions . . . superstitiously adopted and obstinately adhered to, as in the days of *Aristotle*'.

Not only silly and superstitious, she might be 'too far from proper advice, or unable to pay for it' and so prey to the 'dangerous abuse of powerful medicines' for, at the *critical time of life*, the female sex are often visited with various diseases of the *chronic kind*: I have observed, *more women die about this age*, than at any other period, during the years of maturity'. And, he suggested, it is almost entirely due to her character if she suffers like this. Some women he has treated,

who have lived temperately, and are naturally very
healthy, escape without much inconvenience; and I have
known some delicate women inclined to *hysterics*, and
nervous disorders, who were relieved by this change, and
became much more strong and healthy than before; whilst
others, on the contrary, of a sanguine disposition, who
used little exercise, and indulged their appetites to excess,
often suffered severely at this juncture [and] are subject to
pain and giddiness of the head, hysteric disorders, colic
pains, and a female weakness . . . piles, stranguary, itchi-
ness, rheumatism, scurvy, obstructions of the glands, low
spirits and melancholy . . . or the most grievous and distressing of all human maladies, *cancerous tumours* of the breast
and womb.

Whilst piling on the terrible consequences of a life of indulgence
and fancy, Leake does admit that 'it may appear extraordinary
that so many disorders should happen from a change so usual
with every female.' But in his view it was transgression and
disobedience to the laws of nature through the 'many excesses
introduced by luxury, and the irregularity of the passions'
which determined whether a woman would suffer badly at the
menopause or not. This is the physician as moral arbiter – an
increasingly popular, authoritarian stance.[17]

Both Leake and Manning agreed that at menopause 'the
uterus becomes hard and vessels collapse [and all] returns to
almost the same state as before the years of puberty'; that
with a

dissipation of the blood and juices, and the consequent
emptiness, and rigidity of their vessels, they will gradually
shrink up and contract; so that instead of the wonted

freshness and smoothness of the skin when replete with moisture; age and wrinkles, those unwelcome intruders, will come at last.

It was imperative to make sure any cessation of bleeding was natural rather than an untimely or unnatural stoppage, though how a physician could properly ascertain this is not clear. What he could do was promote bleeding with leeches and a knife 'once a month, more or less copiously, as occasion may require', a purgative which 'will be necessary; and may be continued a considerable time with great safety and advantage', a 'spare and simple diet of vegetables, fish and "spoon meats", light white wines diluted with water, or toast and water only', to 'increase exercise to aid perspiration' and, if she is 'delicate and subject to a female weakness, night sweats, or an habitual purging, with flushings in the face and a hectic fever', then she should have 'ass's milk, jellies, London Porter, or a glass of rhenish wine' at meals. Twice a day she should have a 'tea-cup full of a restorative infusion' and when she is stronger 'she may venture on sea-bathing, or the cold bath' or, failing all this, just 'leave the rest to nature'.[18]

Menopausal women who had led an unnatural life of vanity and grossness could be 'seized with acute or chronic diseases, of which they die'. The physician William Buchan stated clearly that 'women of gross habit, at this period of life, have ulcerous sores break out on their ancles, or in other parts of the body' because fluids were suppressed and unable to freely leave the body. Buchan's terrible warnings were contained in his *Domestic Medicine: or, a Treatise on the prevention and cure of Diseases by Regimen and Simple Medicines* (1772), a comprehensive work written for the public, an early medical compendium for family use which he 'endeavoured to make plain and useful . . . utility is the aim'. Women, he begins in his apparently straightforward fashion, start to menstruate at 'about the age of fifteen, and leave it off about fifty, which renders these two periods the most critical of their lives'. Utility with an alarming touch of anxiety. Warming to his theme, he continues, 'That period of life at which the *Menses* cease to flow, is . . . very critical to the sex. The stoppage of any customary evacuation, however small, is sufficient to disorder the whole frame, and often to destroy life itself', as women either 'fall into chronic disorders, or die about this time'. His grim picture is alleviated by the idea that 'such of them however as survive it, without contracting any chronic disease often become more healthy and hardy than they were before, and enjoy strength and vigour to a very great age'. Moderate living was his prescription. Should the '*Menses* cease all of a sudden, in women of a full habit', then they 'ought to abate somewhat of their usual quantity of food, especially of the more nourishing kind, as flesh, eggs, etc. They ought likewise to take sufficient exercise, and to keep the body open.' He suggests a bowl of rhubarb once or twice a week. Management and common sense remained the prevailing options for any discomforts menopausal women might experience. As Penelope Aubin on the life of *Lady Lucy* (1739) put it, 'such a Change of Life must occasion a strange Alteration in a short Time'. Opiates might provide welcome respite or escape from life's trials generally, but these drugs came with acknowledged difficulties.[19]

John Fothergill's remarkably sensible and clear essay 'Of the management proper at the cessation of the menses' (1774) recognized that the only legitimate help a physician could give was good advice on palliative care.[20] Fothergill had

written his essay on the menopause for the benefit of inexperienced physicians consulted by older female patients:
evidence that women themselves were part of the medical
appropriation of the menopause. A Yorkshireman born of a
substantial Quaker family (his father, a lay-preacher, had
travelled extensively, visiting America three times between
1706 and 1737), he was apprenticed in 1728 to an eminent
apothecary, bookseller, botanist and Quaker minister. In 1734
he went to Edinburgh to study medicine. When he became a
practising physician he opposed prevailing treatments and
was credited with saving many lives. His success strengthened his medical practice and, although he never held a
hospital or court appointment, he soon became one of the
wealthiest physicians in England. He wrote on tic douloureux
(sometimes called Fothergill's disease), migraine, angina
pectoris, epilepsy, *hydrocephalus internus* (tubercular meningitis),
coffee, rabies and obesity, as well as menopause. He became
a respected political adviser to the Quaker members of
the Pennsylvania assembly who sent Benjamin Franklin to
London in 1757. On arrival Franklin fell ill and became
Fothergill's patient, whereupon they became fast friends
and collaborators. When he learned of his death Franklin
wrote, 'I think a worthier man never lived.'

The fact that women were 'taught to look [upon the
menopause] with some degree of anxiety' – just as they are
today – vexed Fothergill. Unlike most of his medical contemporaries, he appears to have had an impressive empathy
for the menopausal woman, whom he viewed as a sentient
being rather than a slightly infuriating pet. 'The various and
absurd opinions,' he wrote, 'propagated through successive
ages, have tended to embitter the hours of so many a sensible
woman . . . she is naturally alarmed.' The menopause was

not dangerous in itself, he maintained, not a 'morbid' event or a 'disease' as such, it was 'absolutely exempt, in itself, of any inconvenience' and not 'as fatal for the women as is commonly assumed [for] great numbers of women in whom the menstrual discharge ceases' do not perceive 'any alteration in their usual health'. Fothergill doubted whether any of the diseases commonly attributed to menopause were actually part of that syndrome. He thought they might be just coincidental to it and if so, the paradoxical image of a natural process carrying innumerable serious ailments became almost incomprehensible.

An ethical man, aware and unafraid of the limitations of his profession, he had 'reasonable confidence that, with very little aid, Nature is sufficient to provide for her own security on this occasion'. He was part of a new breed of godfearing Nonconformists, the industrial 'aristocracy', often Quakers like himself, and they accepted that a natural phenomenon needed little treatment, only management. He eschewed the prevailing practices of bleeding and purging, and employed diet, cordials, clean air and Fothergill's Pill to strengthen women who came to him with menopausal complaints. He prescribed the popular remedies that women recommended to each other and produced a preparation of antimony, aloes, scammony and colocynth, a bestseller for over a century. Emollient words calmed any unnecessary fears and instilled confidence in his ability to nullify the alleged ghastly effects of the menopause, while a practical, common-sense regime focused the mind and the body. This was the basis of his great success and lasting influence.

There was a growing market for 'secret' purgatives and uterine drops against disorders 'that most women labour under, when being between forty and fifty years', including

'Pills of Rufus', 'Pills of Franck', a 'sacred tincture' and an
'*élixir de propriété*' containing purgatives such as aloe and poly-
chrest to evacuate morbid matter or restart menstruation.
The medical profession recognized gynaecology as a specialization and played an increasing role in the medical care of, in
the main, wealthy upper-class women. But there is no evidence that the frequency or severity of the menopause
increased during the eighteenth century.[21]

In France a translation of Fothergill's ('*le célèbre praticien de
Londres*') work was published and much praised in 1812. The
expertise of French *accoucheurs* (midwives), their use of forceps
and specula, their devotion to their patients and their lucid
exposition of their ideas had gained them, and by extension the
medical profession, a new measure of trust. But there was disquiet over 'the unknown *maux secrets*, secret ills, of women'
being exposed by the medical profession, and French physicians' attitude to menopausal women as '*des reines detrônées*',
dethroned queens, who had lost their subjects, admirers,
power and lovers, was a little too overblown for the British
sensibility. Worse, as a Dr Longrois wrote in 1787, the French
believed 'the maxim that nature is the best healer of women in
the climacteric, as, indeed, ailing women at any time is as
false as it is heartless. Nature can heal only simple ills, due to
fortuitous physical causes. Women's maladies are, however,
always complex – affected by their sensitivity and their mental
state.'[22]

Lone voices expressed dissent in France. The philosopher
Jean-Jacques Rousseau (1712–78), who exhorted his country-
men to return to nature, believed that most of people's ills
were of their own making, though he also thought there
was 'no parity between man and woman as to the importance of sex. The male is only a male at certain moments; the

female all her life, or at least throughout her youth [and] is incessantly reminded of her sex.'[23] A woman's life revolved around her womb and dictated a natural, industrious, rural life, eating simple foods, lacking any indulgence in erotic passions, without frustrations, and fulfilling her destiny as a mother. Maurice Chaslon, in his *Essai sur la menstruation* (Paris, 1804), also believed woman to be her womb and adhered to the old idea of the uterus as an irritable, unpredictable and highly sensitive organ, but he disagreed that it almost wilfully carried on polluting and poisoning a woman's system after her menopause was over. He thought women were 'freed from a troublesome and now perfectly useless function (and one sees them, so to speak, return to life and enjoy a new existence)'. Post-menopausal women were more vigorous in their body and temperament and could enjoy a 'pleasant embonpoint, blooming colours, a perfect health [to] replace the langours, the torments, all the ills that a sometimes disorderly and painful menstruation made them experience'.[24] Maurice's voice, sadly, was a lonely if optimistic one.

The first popular 'guidebooks' for menopausal women were written, and sold fast. The burgeoning medical establishment, with a healthier population of its own making, took readily to medicating general life events, such as the menopause. They were creating a disease from a discomfort – a process which often involves stigmatization, and attitudes and assumptions about the menopause proliferated: 'the malady of the women of forty' was a phrase physicians used to describe the 'traumatic' experience of women who painfully realized that the male gaze might be directed at younger women, while they were left with 'cold respect' and 'forced politeness'. This, they agreed, explained women's 'ill-natured, restless, and often agitated' demeanour and the 'terrible harm' that 'merciless time' did.[25] Insights into the female experience of the menopause were rare, though some letters do exist. In 1730 a 46-year-old mother of fourteen children wrote to a professor of the medical faculty in Paris asking for advice. Her periods had been repeatedly delayed, her health so far not deranged except for some slight lassitude and dejection, but 'wishing to escape the troublesome consequences of my age', she wanted him to advise her 'how I must conduct myself in this situation'. At the age of forty-seven Mme de Graffigny wrote to a female friend in October 1742 and described a painful sensation in her left breast. She feared cancer, but when her right breast began to hurt as well she and her physician agreed that 'this is not a cancer, but one of those accidents which correspond to the critical time which, it seems, I am approaching'. Bloodletting had shown her blood to be of poor quality so she decided to 'take little remedies to restore it, if that is possible'. Revealing her anxieties, she wrote, 'Surely I will experience something new every day. Only patience, regimen, and cautions can save me.' Her physician told her 'more or less, which conduct is necessary' and she followed his advice to avoid the effects of 'a step that, as you know, I have feared for a long time'. She was surprised, after all her fear and precautions, when all she experienced was just a little dizziness.

The Swiss physician Samuel Auguste Tissot reported on a patient in 1773 whose periods stopped at the age of forty-four with only some irregular bleeding over a few weeks. Hoping 'that there would be no consequences', she still took 'all the precautions one has to take in this case'. Another woman in 1778 with light, irregular periods suffered a sensation of fiery heat rising to her head, reddening her face, and of profuse sweating and coldness some twenty times a day. She asked for 'a rule of conduct' in this 'only epoch in my life that I fear. For, to die is nothing, but the ills that bring a slow death are horrible and many women succumb to them.' All these women were wealthy and familiar with the ministrations of physicians, so appear to have more menopausal complaints than their rural, less well-off sisters. They exposed themselves to irritations and indulgences, they employed servants and lacked industry, they read novels and frequented theatres, masturbated and were sexually indulgent, ate rich foods, drank coffee, wine and spirits; they even, curse them, breathed bad air. All this unrelenting, self-inflicted stimulation brought them terrible suffering at menopause.[26] It could, of course, be prevented with the physician's advice over long years and with complete acceptance of his authority, drugs, therapies and strictly regulated regimes.

The medical historian Edward Shorter gives the subject of the menopause the most casual and tangential of glances in *A History of Women's Bodies* (1984).[27] It is as though he, too, takes his cue from the physicians of the past in imagining a woman's body is of no concern when she has ceased to reproduce. His history is concerned only with the fecund female body and the menopause gets its paltry mention in a discussion of uterine cancer in older women, when the disease caused them to bleed again. One such woman, who fell ill at the age of seventy-seven, said, 'she had not been in such a state . . . for these last thirty years'. Shorter agrees with an eighteenth-century surgeon that this is the worst of all the 'calamities' to beset 'a sex that seems destined to support the largest share of human misery'. He sees the female body as a reproductive machine, a reservoir of sickness and dysfunction, and a 'victimized' entity. Women, he argues, are 'vulnerable to their own bodies . . . Their inferior status in [past] centuries resulted in some measure, from their victimization by their reproductive organs in a way that men have not been victimized.' Shorter surmises that women complied voluntarily with patriarchy because they felt themselves deeply debased and humiliated by the gynaecological afflictions that were their lot all along.[28]

Some historians still understand women as historically passive and impotent, and – resurrecting Aristotelian notions of the perfect male body (as though biology doesn't affect men and their bodies) and the much less than perfect female body – defective or deformed. And if we erroneously entertain the idea of women victimized by their own nature and as 'direct victims of male sexuality', where does that leave the actions and beliefs of society, of the medical profession, religion, politics and economics? It is difficult, if not impossible, to read authors such as Shorter without being forcibly struck by a not always subtle, but always present, misogyny. The shame, contempt and confusion that shrouded diseases peculiar to women were extremely hard to dislodge, rooted as they were in fundamental ideas about the very nature of things. The ruthless, sometimes rancorous age of medical reform which was beginning to colonize the bodies and functions of women rested on the negative assumptions of the past. As the menopause was transformed from a natural phenomenon into a disease, this aspect of medicine became a form of purgatory for older women.

4

ON THE BORDERLAND
OF PATHOLOGY

Most women are not quite normal

James Compton Burnett, *The Change of Life in Women*

Menopausal and post-menopausal women languished in a medical no-man's-land of sexual and social limbo. The swelling band of gynaecologists, having inherited Hippocratic ideas of the female body and its reproductive role, reinforced that middle-aged women were neither truly feminine nor truly masculine. Neither one thing nor the other, they were worryingly unstable in mind and body. Prey to volatile appetites, women might newly discover a desire for sex. And having acquired some of the male's guarded autonomy, a woman became an increasingly ambivalent figure. Released from the tyranny of reproduction, who knew what she might demand for herself and others like her? Better she consumed herself than those around her.

Cornelia Bandi, aged sixty-two, was recorded in the *Annual*

Register, 1763, as having been mysteriously reduced to soot, ash and bone in her own home. Her body was discovered as a heap of ashes, her legs and arms untouched, with fatty, foetid moisture clinging to the furniture, tapestries and walls, penetrating the drawers and dirtying the linen. Twenty years earlier the burning of sixty-year-old Grace Pitt had been described in the *Transactions of the Royal Society of London*. Consumed by flames, Pitt was found by her daughter, who tried to save her by throwing water over the fire. It is recorded that Pitt 'had drunk a large quantity of spirituous liquor'. Mary Clues, a widow, appeared in the register ten years later similarly incinerated. She had been 'much addicted to intoxication' following the death of her husband and was found after her neighbours saw smoke issuing from her bedroom window. Little remained of her and what did was 'entirely calcined, and covered with a whitish efflorescence. The people were much surprised that the furniture had sustained so little injury.' Pierre-Aimé Lair (1769–1853) summed up the deaths of such women beyond their prime with a rhetoric of revulsion:

Young persons, distracted by other passions, are not much addicted to drinking; but when love, departing along with youth, leaves a vacuum in the mind, if its place be not supplied by ambition or interest, a taste for gaming, or religious fervour, it generally falls a prey to intoxication. This passion still increases as the others diminish, especially in women, who can indulge it without restraint . . . It may have been observed that the obesity of women, as they advance in life, renders them more sedentary . . . Dancing and walking, which form salutary recreation for young persons, are at a certain age interdicted as much by nature as by prejudice. It needs, therefore, excite no astonishment, that old women, who are in general more corpulent and more addicted to drinking, and who are often motionless like inanimate masses, during the moment of intoxication, should experience the effects of combustion.[1]

Young people dancing, so often disapproved of, is praised by Lair compared with indolent, immobile, lumps of pointless, aged female flesh. It would be an outrage if these women had got up to dance. This burning up and destruction is plainly nature's way. Lair's collection of twelve cases of spontaneous combustion, 'Essai sur les combustions humaines produites par un long abus de liqueures spiriteuses', published in the Journal de Physique in 1800, included supporting material by a famous French surgeon, Monsieur Le Cât (1700–68). Papers and reports by well-respected physicians written about these disturbing mortalities in The Annual Register, the Transactions and the Journal de Médecine show that spontaneous human combustion was accepted by the medical community of the time. The inflammable beings were mainly older women, described as sedentary, corpulent and sodden with alcohol. They were useless, vice-ridden and unattractive, and were burned up through the 'viciousness' of their own decaying bodies. They had consumed themselves in a righteous parody of the public burnings of women who not long ago would have been vilified and destroyed as witches.[2]

Lair's work was translated into English and appeared in Tilloch's Philosophical Magazine, later used by Charles Dickens as research for his novel Bleak House (1853). The writer George Henry Lewes (1817–78) criticized the novelist's acceptance of spontaneous human combustion as fact, though Dickens was satisfied by the 'recorded opinions and experiences of distinguished medical professors, French, English, and

Scotch, in more modern days', and he would 'not abandon the facts until there shall have been a considerable Spontaneous Combustion of the testimony'.[3] In letters and in the preface to *Bleak House*, Dickens was adamant that Lewes was quite mistaken

> in supposing the thing to have been abandoned by all authorities . . . before I wrote that description I took pains to investigate the subject. There are about thirty cases on record, of which the most famous, that of the Countess Cornelia de Bandi Cesenate was minutely investigated . . . The appearances beyond all rational doubt observed in that case, are the appearances observed in [the book]. The next most famous instance happened at Rheims . . . and the historian in that case is LE CAT, one of the most renowned surgeons produced by France.

Medical testimony was inviolable it seemed, and even their subjective musings were given substance. In the male gaze, the menopausal, 'unsexed' and manly woman was the least beautiful of her sex. Many confessed themselves confounded by such an apparently masculine and 'unamiable' creature; to men 'an amazon never fails to be forbidding'.[4]

> With the shrinking of the ovaria . . . there is a corresponding change in the outer form . . . the form becomes angular, the body lean, the skin wrinkled. The hair changes in colour and loses its luxuriancy; the skin is less transparent and soft, and the chin and upper lip become downy . . . With this change in the person there is an analogous change in the mind, temper and feelings. The woman approximates in fact to a man, or in one word, she is a *virago* . . . This unwomanly

condition undoubtedly renders her repulsive to man, while
her envious, overbearing temper, renders her offensive to
her own sex.[5]

M. Panckoucke, editor of a dictionary of medical science published in Paris in 1821, included this less than rigorous entry
under 'Femme': 'When the desires of nature are fulfilled,
women gradually lose their bloom, and the delicate flowers
around which all gathered. All men then disappear like the
morning dew.'[6] Proof, were any required, that women were
past regard when no longer fertile, non-beings, almost less
than human. The British anthropologist Alexander Walker
(1783–1853) produced a fallaciously subtle, quasi-scientific
book for the male gaze in which he idealized passive, youthful, fecund female beauty and recoiled, horrified, from any
woman who might approximate any real equality with man.
In the spurious *Beauty: Illustrated Chiefly by an Analysis and
Classification of Beauty in Woman* (London, 1836) he claimed that
his studies of humans and animals explained how 'Beauty,
Health, and Intellect' and 'Deformity, Disease, and Insanity'
were passed on through the generations and, not only this,
he emphatically reinforced woman's alleged inferiority
through his vision of nature's design. Walker's theories were
influential and many believed that his observations could be
put to good use in 'selecting the fit progenitors of our race'.
In his work *Intermarriage*, Walker maintained that woman has
a larger reproductive system than man, so it must follow
that this dictates women's function, both natural and social:
'It is with these vital and reproductive organs and functions
that the whole life of woman is associated . . . all that is
connected with love is far more essential to woman than to
man.' In comparison, 'the cerebral, or organ of the will, is

small in women.' These are 'statements of truth' according to Walker, who warned that it would be extremely dangerous for mankind to neglect the apparently obvious lessons of anatomy and physiology.

A young and fecund woman, in Walker's subjectively unscientific opinion, was literally 'encased in beauty', especially her 'posterior . . . unquestionably the *chef d'oeuvre* of nature'. Her delicate tissues, suppleness and the 'soft parts' of her composition all 'indicate very clearly the passive state to which nature has destined woman'. But the woman whose ovaries were 'inert' was akin 'in forms and habits to men'. She may, for example, display a 'partial growth of a beard . . . in the decline of life', she sometimes undergoes 'remarkable modifications' in that 'her neck swells . . . her voice assumes another expression; her moral habits totally change'. Such unpleasant incipient manliness had reinforcing parallels in nature for, he argues, 'the same general principle [occurs in] female birds, when they have ceased to lay eggs [they] occasionally assume the plumage, and, to a certain extent, the other characters of the male'.

Walker's analysis did allow for exceptions and if the physical form did not suddenly deteriorate and fat was allowed to accumulate 'in the cellular tissue under the skin and elsewhere . . . this effaces any wrinkles which might have begun to furrow the skin, rounds the outlines anew, and again restores an air of youth and freshness'. Women who were so fortunate as to put on a couple of pounds could experience 'the age of return'. So all was not lost as long as she was 'otherwise favourably organized'. She might then develop a 'majestic air' which, if she was lucky, 'still interests for a number of years'. When her time was up all she would have left to cling to 'amidst these ruins' was the 'entireness of the hair' and this, along with her placidity, amiable countenance, and 'caressing manners and charming graces' could, at a pinch, 'almost make us [men] forget youth and beauty'.[7] Her value was measured only by her perceived attractiveness to men – particularly Walker himself, one suspects.

Lest the reader be suspicious of Walker's agenda – suspicions aroused perhaps by the twenty-two shadowy plates of naked female specimens arranged in various coyly classical poses and toying unconsciously with gauzey drapes – he reiterates that the work was published 'in relation to decency, morals, progeny, function, determination of parentage'. All that dwelling on the '*chef d'oeuvres* of nature' was in the interests of function and procreation, for 'be it known that the critical judgment and pure taste for beauty are the sole protection against low and degrading connexions'.[8] His cloying sentimentality barely disguised the hypocrisy and brutality of his words.

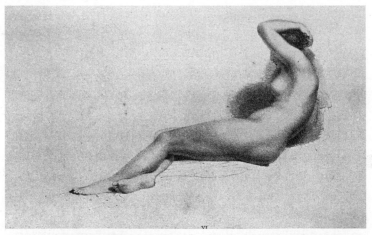

Alexander Walker titillates his fellow men with the ideal young and passive female – before she reaches menopause and becomes unpleasantly, stridently 'manly'.

The American physician Charles Meigs, lecturing to his medical students in 1848, asked them to imagine what on earth a menopausal woman had to expect other than 'grey hairs, wrinkles [and] the gradual decay of these physical or personal attractions, which heretofore have commanded the flattering image of society'. With a real and ghastly pleasure in his descriptive language he taught his eager young men that:

> The pearls of the mouth are become tarnished, the hay-like odour of the breath is gone, the rose has vanished from the cheek, and the lily is no longer the vain rival of the forehead or the neck. The dance is preposterous, and the throat no longer emulates the voice of the nightingale. All these are melancholy convictions, and not even the arguments of Tully, in his Treatise on Old Age, can drive away the painful truth or make wrong the better reason.[9]

What contempt and loathing there are in his words. While ostensibly dispelling the 'aura of anxiety surrounding middle age which [he] believed stemmed from an ill-informed and misleadingly negative stereotype of the effects of the change of life circulating amongst the general public', he drove home the misconceptions further and compounded the negativity directed at menopausal and post-menopausal women.[10]

Older women who did not conform to the conventional passive, asexual role assigned to them were the legitimate butt of jeers and scorn. Older men were occasionally subjected to a similar brand of scorn, but an old man in love with a younger woman was accorded greater sympathy than an older woman yearning to love and be loved. No change there then. Women were mercilessly lampooned, often as a ludicrous Dame who still has two ever-present characteristics: she is thoroughly middle-aged and is very plain, at the very least a parody of her youthful self if not downright hideous. In the theatre, in the music-hall and in pantomime, men playing the manly-woman could get away with greater and riskier larks. They were caricatures of a caricature; their make-up was a mask of femininity and youth, all their actions were outrageously slapstick, and their role was the 'animated comic valentine'. Often displaying a quick, cruel and capricious temper, Dames portrayed older women as shrewish, with an absurd love of flattery and, of course, a tendency to feel unrequited and inappropriate passion for young men. Guilty of a ludicrous dependence on the disguising powers of cosmetics and false hair, they bring to mind George Saville's gushing young girls of fifty and Swift's decrepit 'nymph'. The spiteful rhyme *A Pretty Little Alphabet for Pretty Little Ladies* spelt out the error of their ways:

> D is for dye used to turn her curls red;
> E is her ear which is wax as a dolly's;
> F is the fashion, which prompts all these follies;

> T is the false teeth that she shows when she talks;
> U's unreality – bane of the age;
> V the vain feeling that makes it the rage . . .[11]

Augustus Gardner's *Conjugal Sins: Against the Laws of Life and Health and Their Effects Upon the Father, Mother, and Child* (New York, 1870) noted that 'the body itself does not long delay entering into decrepitude, and soon we see the woman once so favoured by nature when she was charged with the duty of reproducing the species degraded to the level of a being who has no further duty to perform in the world'. Books like this, on 'hygiene', became very popular, with titles such as *How To Grow Handsome* (New York, 1890) – not beautiful, of course, now that she is a manly woman that would be asking too much.

A woman who didn't regard her sex life as dictated by biology and beauty was Amandine Aurore Lucile Dupin, Baronne Dudevant, the nineteenth-century novelist George Sand (1804–76). She took a young lover when she was in her late sixties, a vigorous painter she called the 'Mastodon'. One of her literary peers and friends, Gustave Flaubert, wrote to her suggesting she 'act her age' but she replied with feeling, 'And what, you want me to stop loving?' Her unconventional life aroused very different responses in men; she was thought of as the most womanly woman but also as stupid, heavy, garrulous and immoral.

Some women writers approached their ageing sisters with derision. During the *belle époque* books on beauty were often written by titled women for the married and middle-aged of their sex. Perfection was defined by the Baroness d'Orchamps and the Countess de Tramar as 'health, freshness, velvety smooth unwrinkled skin' and a svelte figure. They advised women over forty to forge a 'career of beauty' by fighting the 'defects' of age and blossoming into 'an opulent, captivating flower'. Mme Lucas, who opened the first beauty 'institute' in Paris in 1895, said that 'a woman can and should be loved until she is seventy-five . . . To love and be loved, you must be a flower. I am the horticulturalist of women.' Gardening metaphors aside, older women were told that they should continue in their efforts to please men, be the 'most complete instrument of voluptuousness', and be vigilantly lovely if they were to keep these apparently flighty men by their sides.

This 'supreme disaster for femininity' is an old ruse, based on fear, and it was fuelled by the French medical profession's greater interest in the menopause.[12] French case studies of menopause collected by Adam Raciborski in the 1860s were still being cited in the 1930s, with all the cultural assumptions of the past intact. The German doctor Bernhard Bauer wrote in his book *Woman* (1927) that 'the mind of the old woman is as unattractive as her appearance', but the American William J. Fielding thought that 'many women are more attractive at fifty than they were at twenty-five; and . . . they may be more charming at sixty than they were at thirty'. Eliza Farnham's lonely voice extolled the lasting beauty of women as 'the register of value in development, a record of Experience, whose legitimate office is to perfect the life, a legible language to those who will study it, of the majestic mistress, the soul'. And Dr Elizabeth Sloan Chesser mused on the idea 'that women age sooner than men, but this seems to me one of those popular superstitions born of masculine vanity'.

Ovid wrote in *Ars Amatoria* that 'the woman whose youth is past, including her whose hair is grey, is a good field for seeding'. At this age, he mused, 'women are particularly clever in love'. Byron, in *Don Juan*, says that 'the young woman ignores the elements and especially the nuances of love' and 'in her maturity only does she comprehend what it is and what it requires'. The 'preference which some men feel for women who are in full maturity is well known. Some women confess that it is in this age they obtain the maximum degree of sexual success.' The French historian Jules Michelet, when he himself was sixty, was commenting on a woman who had 'entered upon this decline' yet who complains that her character and intellect are not given sufficient attention because her face is a little faded. Missing her point spectacularly he, too, fails to address her character and intellect, dwelling solely on how youthful 'plastic beauty' is transformed into 'sexual beauty': 'If the face is faded, does that say that the flesh is less firm? In these cases not rarely is the body twenty-five while the face is forty. There are wrinkles around the eyes and on the cheeks, it is true. But usually, the knees and elbows previously angular, now show pretty dimples.' Michelet has been described as an essential figure in European historiography, renowned for his research into 'patterns of ingrained coherence in nature' in which he combined anthropology, political science, ethics and history.[13] Gregorio Marañón (1887–1960), an influential physician and philosopher who founded the Institute of Medical Pathology in Madrid and was president of the Institute of Experimental Endocrinology and the Institute of Biological Research, suggested that grey hair could coincide with 'an energetic and lasting ovarian function'. It might also herald a tendency to sexual inversion or 'menopausal virilism', by which he meant lesbianism. These women would develop a robustness, a deep voice, an 'altered psychic state', and an energy and aggressiveness they did not have before, and it was 'much more frequent than supposed' by Freud and other psychologists.[14] He may have visited the music-halls, too, because he knew that the 'most common people personify this transformation in the physical and psychical type of "the mother-in-law"'.

New, scientific medicine was behaving as culture and tradition demanded, in its eagerness to instil disgust and fear of mortal dangers and of physical and psychological disease in women. If she was hobbled by anxiety, what could she hope to achieve? Kept busy worrying about and fighting her mind, body and inclinations, she had little or no time and energy to struggle against any external injustice or prejudice. The physician dealt with women through a distorted lens, her sensations and peculiarities were viewed in the light of prevailing cultural constraints, and medical assumptions were awarded the status of 'scientific' truth. This was symptomatic of the nineteenth-century drive for medical professionalization, and the publication of new medical journals, with a larger, more critically concerned professional and public understanding, began to formalize theories, treatments and attitudes. Most medical careers and reputations were built on deferential and personal attendance on patients, particularly the precious wealthy ones.[15] Before the medical registration measures of 1858 there were no precise parameters to the term 'qualified medical practitioner', and the struggle for professional status inevitably included the designation and categorization of diseases to legitimize the orthodox physicians' claims. Growing specialization led to the development of newly distinct branches of medical sciences, including neurology and psychology which had arisen initially from the traditional duality of mind and body: the view that human nature was both somatopsychic and psychosomatic.[16]

In this febrile atmosphere of reform a 'doctrine of crisis' was employed to describe the gynaecological life of women and was firmly linked to various nervous disorders, especially hysteria. The 'hysterization' of women's bodies was enhanced by the greater sensitivity thought to be a desirable feminine characteristic and moral virtue.[17] The unreliability of the minds and bodies of women became medical fact and a series of worrying, possibly fatal, crisis-inspired new technologies were developed with increasingly rigid controls, to bring female instability under control. If they were prone to so many diseases, women might also infect the male, so pills, potions, constraints and taboos followed.[18] The physician carved out for himself a privileged view of the female body, inside and out, jealously guarding the right to see and know what was traditionally, ordinarily and most modestly kept hidden. The power of this medical gaze, its penetrating and apparent understanding, infused with power and supporting a moral and behavioural superstructure of thoughtful senti-mentality over brute realism, seemed almost mystical, or magical, to the uninitiated.

The culmination of the female 'thirty-year pilgrimage' through her sexual life — as if it most definitely ended here — was now, if not the advertised 'gateway to death', almost uni-versally and popularly seen as the back door to uselessness. The American manufacturer W. R. Greg, in a piece entitled 'Why women are redundant' (1862), damned 'hundreds and thousands of women . . . who, not having the natural duties and labours of wives and mothers', were so obviously with-out value. Those who no longer 'undertake the special functions of the sex are of secondary importance', opined the paleontol-ogist Edward Cope in a politically charged and defamatory piece entitled 'The relation of the sexes to government', pub-lished in *Popular Science Monthly* in 1888. Menopausal and post-menopausal women were utterly insignificant, without any physical, intellectual or social purpose. Any mental, emotional or bodily strains that women felt at mid-life were taken as the signs of menopause and wholly equated with crisis, even though women lived through it and, in general, lived on for longer than men, and in better health. Life expectancy was similar for middle-class white English and American women at the end of the nineteenth century, estimated at 51.08 years, compared with male life expectancy of *c.* 48.23 years.[19]

During the second half of the nineteenth century a sub stantial number of works covering the menopause or devoted particularly to it were published. Thomas Laycock's treatise *The Morbid Phenomena of Menopause* (1840) set the grim scene and discussed post-menopausal women in terms of their virtue: 'there is less of passion, less disappointment, less mortified vanity, and fewer causes for indulgence in evil tempers and foolish caprices'. Love, ordered Charles Menville de Ponsan, must be 'banished forever from their hearts' as 'only the product of imagination, and not the manifestation of a true need, provoked by nature in the interests of procreation'. He recommended women abstain from sex completely if over forty, as even the mere thought of sex would irritate the uterus and draw forth blood towards it. Her 'submission' would be rewarded by good health and tranquil happiness, and the slightest transgression would be 'severely punished' – whether by Charles or by nature is not made clear. The loss of erotic feeling and attention would be amply compensated for, he wrote consolingly, by the pleasures of domestic life.[20] In the medical mind a woman was her sexual and reproductive function and very little else. This is where her value and virtue lay, and her later peculiarities made her so different as to be almost another species, an object of fascination and revulsion.

The spectacle of women's physical 'decline' was as much of a preoccupation as ever. In 1841 the physician Michael Ryan described how they apparently withered and swelled at the same time. As 'the peculiarities of women cease, the breasts collapse, the skin shrivels, the cheeks and neck wither, the eyes recede in their sockets, they become remarkably corpulent'. George Corfe, in *Man and His Many Changes or, Seven Times Seven* (1849), detailed the 'degeneration, at the climacteric period of life [which] gradually and insensibly comes on'. Women 'grow fat, with shortness of breath, attended by a pale, flabby skin . . . fat now takes the place of muscles, glands, and even bones'. More frighteningly, 'diseased growths not infrequently present themselves about this eventful period of life, and tend to destroy the healthy parts around them'. Those 'women of riper years . . . who possess intelligent minds' were in greater danger still, for they had time and imagination to dwell on their decline and they suffered 'very humiliating' and 'strange attacks'. These 'seizures are not wholly wilful, neither are they wholly uncontrollable', but were due to 'sedentary habits' which have induced 'sluggishness of liver and weak digestion', and could 'merge into a misanthropical state'.[21] Indeed, according to the obstetrician Samuel Ashwell (1798–1852), any menopausal ills arise 'from the fact, that nature and health are often sacrificed to fashion and luxury' and 'are attributable not to necessity, but mainly to habits, unwisely begun, and still more unwisely continued'.[22]

Women, then, were instructed to live 'appropriately' for there was 'scarcely any organ or part of the body . . . which may not suffer . . . as the direct or remote consequence of this great change'. Ashwell acknowledged a 'universal impression that organic maladies, especially of the breast and uterus, are more likely to take place at this than at any other time', but doubted whether the menopause, 'as it is a natural process, has anything to do with their original production'. Though he certainly thought that the 'derangement' and, in line with ancient thought, any 'superfluity of blood with no accurate outlet' could lead to cancer. Sounding like an advocate of the modern-day spa weekend, he suggested women might try a mustard hip-bath, pediluvia or, better still, frictions with stimulating embrocations. At any rate, what was recommended was an attempt to maintain the norm of menstruation, with 'encouragement, by any gentle means, of the catamenial flow'. Women were to expect 'injurious consequences . . . if menstruation is suppressed, as it is habitual and necessary'; they themselves called it 'the critical or dodging time' or 'the turn of life, etc.' So far, so traditionally terrifying, but Ashwell, though not admitting his lack of real knowledge, even though it was 'impossible to provide any precise information', went on to say that it must not be 'supposed, that the effect of these great changes is always morbid'; he had known of 'several patients thus dealt with, who never had afterwards one hour's inconvenience'. All these women were, of course, 'aware that such symptoms may be expected to occur, and they are in consequence alive to their approach', and a 'timidity, a dread of sudden disease, irritability of temper, a disposition to seclusion, impaired appetite and broken sleep with physical weakness and inquietude, are common indications'. Modesty allowing, most of these fearful but physically healthy women could still, he thought, be convinced of an examination: 'they will readily yield if . . . safety be urged as their justification', as though their yielding were some kind of illicit seduction.

Physical examinations came into play early in the nineteenth century and enabled modern scientific medicine to pre-empt disease and attack it if it were discovered. Physicians might now be able to do more than just manage symptoms. Traditionally a sick person would have related details of their complaint, telling the physician about their regime – diet, bowel motions, emotional upsets, sleeping habits – and expected a diagnosis on this basis. The physician, using his experience and observation, would weigh up the information and examine carefully, by eye, the demeanour and appearance of his patient, rarely touching him or her except to take the pulse; he might look at the tongue, sniff bad odours and listen to coughs and wheezes. Too much touching was possibly suspect to both parties and thought undignified and indelicate. There were no diagnostic tools to assist the senses; stethoscopes and similar instruments did not appear until after 1800 and were often strongly resisted, particularly the speculum. Queen Victoria's last physician, Sir James Reid, recorded that he didn't attend the Queen's bedside until she was on her death-bed, and it wasn't until she had died that he discovered she had suffered from a 'ventral hernia, and a prolapse of the uterus', revealing that he had never given her a full physical examination.[23]

It could not be denied, wrote Ashwell, that women 'often have sufficient reason for their anxieties', especially where such delicacy prevailed. At menopause, 'the extinction of this extraordinary excretion' and the death of the reproductive faculty were an event that heralded 'magnitude in the life of a woman'. Samuel Mason agreed, declaring that 'women dread this period', and any women that read any of these works might have thought rightly so.[24] Lay and medical opinion agreed that this 'crisis' lessened rational responsibility, and the 'disturbed organic and physical functions' accounted for deviant behaviour at 'the menopausis epoch'.[25] Nineteenth-century female suicide peaked at menopause. A study of 198 female suicides at the end of the century observed that seventy-seven of them were aged between forty and fifty years. A 41-year-old woman, S. de L., who was married but had no children, was said to have led a very tranquil and religious life. Living '*happily* in her calm surroundings, she shocked her relatives and all who knew her' by drinking poison. She 'left no note . . . Yet it was known that *menstruation*, never very active, *had been absent two months*.'[26] If the value of women rested on their reproductive function then the menopause heralded a terrible loss of meaning, security and power.

For John Robertson, whose *Essays and Notes on the Physiology and Diseases of Women, and on Practical Midwifery* was published in London in 1851, motherhood occupied a short period of a woman's life, showing that nature did not limit her role to reproducing and nurturing. Continuation of life post-menopause proved to him that:

> Woman is destined to other duties than belong to the mere animal; that her day is not to close when the offices of mother and nurse have been fulfilled, but rather than now, when ripe in knowledge and experience, it remains for her to *train* those to whom she has given birth . . . herself, mean-while, continuing to shed on domestic society that benign, humanizing influence, which her moral constitution, when purified and elevated by Christian religion, is so eminently fitted to exercise.[27]

She was not finished at menopause but should endeavour to live a life circumscribed by Christian 'domestic society'.

Female sexuality was not understood as being independent from the male's, revolving as it did around pregnancies, childbirth, nursing, family care and menopausal 'anxieties'. Men's sexuality was defined, in popular and medical litera-ture, as instrumental, forceful and direct, whilst women's was supposedly expressive and responsive, and medical dis-coveries were used to validate conventional ideas about femininity and women's sexuality. That women were natural invalids was almost universally embraced and there was a pervasive belief, even amongst many women, that biology had incapacitated them. In 1892 Dr J. Webster, pontificating on the post-menopausal woman's sexual appetite, thought that in many 'it disappears more or less completely; in some it remains unaltered, while in others it may increase in intensity. There can be little doubt that the first of these variations is to be considered as the most common.' Cases which presented with a 'marked increase' in libido were 'generally due to some abnormal state'. Female sexuality was either non-existent (i.e. in the 'normal' woman) or pathologically, unconscionably male, according to the influential likes of the surgeon William Acton, who wrote *The Functions and Disorders of the Reproductive Organs* (London, 1857), and John Ruskin, the writer, critic and famously life-long celibate.

F. H. Marshall's *Physiology of Reproduction* (1910) placed womankind in its entirety firmly on 'the borderland of pathology'. But in the 1850s Edward Tilt (1815–93) had already smuggled them across the border. His pivotal, influential and exhaustive work, *The Change of Life in Health and Disease. A Practical Treatise on the Nervous and Other Affections Incidental to Women at the Decline of Life* (London, 1857), appeared in Britain and America and was found remarkable for 'the depth of its ideas and, above all, its methodology'. Tilt had trained at St George's Hospital, London, and then Paris, graduating in 1839. During his Parisian studies Tilt had learned about the speculum as an aid to diagnosis and he later encouraged its use in Britain. Settling in London in the 1850s he began specializing in midwifery and the diseases of women, was appointed physician-*accoucheur* to the Farringdon General Dispensary and Lying-in Charity and was one of the original fellows of the Obstetrical Society of London, formed in 1859, eventually being elected its president for 1874–5. Tilt's formidable work was cutting edge, 'a book of the present time', and this when Fothergill's eighty-year-old study on the menopause was still in current use and had just been republished.

Truly a Victorian man of science, Tilt began by clarifying his terms and reifying his chosen disease (and career). It was: 'Climacteria' in Latin; 'Climacteric', 'Change of Life', 'Critical Time' and 'Time of Life' in English; '*Temps Critique*', '*Age de Retour*' and '*Ménopause*' in French; and '*Aufhören die Weiblichen Reinigung*' in German. Wherever you might happen to be geographically, Tilt defined the change of life as the period of time from 'irregularities which precede the last menstrual flow, and end with the re-settlement of health'. The term 'climacteric', meaning a critical period in human life, was, he thought, more usable than 'menopause', which merely and literally means the cessation of bleeding. His was a medical manual for the practising physician, and its chapters took in the general and special pathology of the change which included diseases of the brain, the reproductive organs, the skin, heart and other diseases of 'rare occurrence'. A magnificent catch-all for what is an imprecise phenomenon.

Above all Tilt was attempting to establish a scientific, quantitative base for explaining the menopause phenomenon even whilst putting the case for the physician 'to be at once a divine, a moralist, and a philosopher' because 'his medicines will, in some cases, be of little use'. Using his study of 500 women 'at the c. of life or who had passed it', he produced a comprehensive list of 120 infirmities, subdivided into 'seven distinct modes of suffering'. Women did not take the menopause seriously enough in his opinion and it was 'not unusual [for them] to refer all their extraordinary sensations to "the c. of life", and to consider that, when they have thus accounted for their diseases, they have at the same time cured them; and in this, most medical men . . . seem to be of the same opinion'. There was work to be done and progress to be made. In America, too, medical attitudes to the menopause were, he insisted, remiss, basing his complaint on Meig's opinion that 'too little regard is paid to the dangers of the crisis [and] fatal mutations are attributed to some trivial cause, and the victim passes away . . . and no increase of knowledge . . . stands in the way of the next victim to a management as unwise and as thoughtless'. In Tilt's view medicine had been negligent in its treatment of the menopause, it should buck up its ideas and give it due regard, and he was the man to do it.[28]

In Tilt's ideas and work we can see a double-edged sword poised over the menopausal woman. He wanted medicine to make the menopause worthy of investigation and treatment. Dismissing it and a woman's complaints and fears may mean that a serious illness was not recognized, despite the fact that his profession could do little to alleviate, let alone cure, such diseases. But, once the menopause fell under the microscope of medical investigation it was transformed into a disease itself, with all the consequences, symptoms, treatments and attendant dreads that transformation brings. Tilt tried to take the sting out of the tail by addressing 'those who deny that the c. of life is a critical period, [and] argue as if *critical* meant *fatal*'. 'In medical language,' he wrote, 'crisis means a sudden change for the better or worse' and it leads 'as often to recovery as to death'. Not wanting to put himself out of business, he intends his work to 'forcibly show the evil effects of the c. of life', and reveals that the 'frequency . . . of intense suffering . . . is proved by carefully noting down what has occurred to women at this period'. The book being based on observation of cases, 'because so little is written on the subject', we can see clearly that it is the women who consult the physicians who provide the knowledge rather than the majority of women who have had their menopause without complaint or, at least, without recourse to a physician.

While the menopause might arrive early through shock, 'severe frost', a fall, a fright, grief or with ovarian tumours, it could also be greatly delayed, not arriving sometimes until a woman is in her sixties, seventies or eighties. Tilt gives the examples of a mother who gave birth for the final time at sixty and menstruated until she was eighty, and of a nun who menstruated until she was 103 years old. The reason for their fecundity is given as 'ovarian activity [which is] commensurate with constitutional vigour'. During their 'c. of life' these women, he says, 'have the power of generating a more than usual amount of heat; and often want less clothing, and even in winter leave their doors and windows wide open'. These 'flushes may be considered as cases of pathological blushing', sometimes following a chill, lasting perhaps two to three minutes and varying greatly in number throughout the day. Conflating, or confusing, nature with cultural assumptions, Tilt blithely suggests that 'the occurrence of flushes so late in life is not to be wondered at, for woman has been made a blushing creature'. He does say, though, that he has 'seen the sudden growth of fat coincide with great improvement in health' and that 'those who became fat-bellied were not troubled with nervous symptoms'. This observation tallies with current wisdom which tells us that oestrogens continue to be produced by adipose tissue. But here his observations part company with his inherited and less empirical beliefs: it is the 'nutritive force' of food which converts the retained blood to fat and he argues in favour of bleeding, even though it is 'out of fashion'. If, he reasons, 'nature bled' then this 'system often deserves imitation [and] should not be neglected in the c. of life'.

Purgatives were useful, too, he thought, but the real and best remedy was the powerful narcotic opium, despite a great mistrust of 'the frequency and the extent of its use'. He puts aside these concerns as not warranted by facts, for 'opium is the most certain and powerful of the aids we possess', and he pooh-poohed the caution of other physicians, saying that 'its use is not to be measured timidly by a table of doses, but by fulfilment of the purpose for which it is given'. On a tour of Egypt, Syria and Turkey he had noted a problem of impotence amongst men and recognized its cause as a 'constant use of opium and its anaphrodisiac action' and, as the 'principal source of cerebral disturbance at the c. of life is the irregular stimulus of the reproductive organs, which are no longer relieved by a regular discharge', he deduces that 'in many cases, the systematic use of camphor, lupulin, hyoscyamus, and opium are required'. Other physicians refused to treat women taking opiates or the euphemistically termed 'soothing injections'. Compton Burnett had one patient, 'a maiden lady of forty-three' with 'painful nerves and flushes that have troubled her ever since she changed [who] is much given to sleeping draughts', but he will help her only on the condition she stops taking the drugs, it being 'quite impossible to really cure people who take hypnotics'.[29] But Tilt was sure of himself, arguing for the use of sedatives and recommending rectal application as the most effective method. Morphia salts, laudanum and the proprietary opiate remedies of Dover's Powder and Battley's solution could be put into a 2-ounce India-rubber bottle. This the patient fills up with warm milk, and after screwing on the canula, and anointing it with a little cold cream, it should be gently pushed up the bowel. When this is done, the firm pressure of the bottle by the hand will empty its contents into the bowel; the bottle should then be withdrawn; the mild nature of the fluid, and its small bulk, almost always allow its being retained.

Inappropriate excitement must be controlled at all costs. Tilt was alarmed by the idea of menopausal women drinking alcohol and thought that if they were not given his drugs they would instinctively fly to other stimulants, the poor to porter and gin, the rich to wine and brandy. He recommended belladonna, too, though it could give 'singular hallucinations', and cherry-laurel, lupulin, castor or ambergris, and in later editions of his book he suggested bromides and chloral-hydrate. The 'subtle fumes of camphor' worked particularly well, he thought, seeming to 'spread like an aura over the nervous system . . . the patient feeling as if she could fly'. Tepid baths would alleviate excitement and uncomfortable flushes like a 'gigantic poultice', or more 'tepid water [and] cold applications may be made to the head, and a stream of cold water directed to the abdomen through a vulcanized India-rubber tube'. These constitute the 'chief remedies' but the benefits of good diet, exercise, travel, avoiding 'balls, routs, operas, etc.' were not to be ignored and, importantly, 'sleep is indispensable to the full effect of all other remedies'. Whilst purporting to provide a new and radical take on menopause treatment Tilt is actually reduced to marrying his empirical findings to centuries-old medical advice with the added ingredient of the odd narcotic or two.

There was an all-pervading theme of drug-induced inertia as the passive answer to the menopause.

Drugs could help with unwanted or undesirable sexual urges, too. Camphor was suggested for treating nymphomania in menopausal women, it being another anaphrodisiac acting to correct the 'toxic influence' of the reproductive system on the brain. Nearly everyone agreed that the reproductive organs should 'no longer require their hitherto appropriate stimulus'. Indeed, Tilt says he was repeatedly told by some of his patients that 'a distaste for connexion was the first sign of an approaching change', but that many 'were driven to the verge of insanity by ovario-uterine excitement'. It is possible, Tilt reluctantly admits, that 'a flickering flame gives a final blaze, so in some women, sexual desire is strongest when the reproductive power is about to be extinguished'. But sexual arousal at menopause is just an 'anomalous if not morbid impulse, depending on either neuralgic or inflammatory affections of the genital organs'. Because of this, he thought it 'unreasonable to marry during this period' unless the 'sanction of a medical advisor' had been obtained. The physician should and must rule a woman's private life because what was she if not congenitally diseased? Women who rashly marry at this age, he sniffed, were invariably and dishonestly 'led to the altar by other than sexual motives', or they were old virgins who should have known better, 'besieged fortresses' brought down too late. Sex was not on the cards, nymphomania less so, and Tilt 'would willingly ignore so painful a subject' if only he could, but, he whined contemptuously, the menopausal 'nervous system is so unhinged'. In fact, the effects of all this disturbance of ovarian activity on the mental faculties were of paramount importance and there was 'almost always some amount of confusion and bewilderment, which seems to deprive women of the mental endowments to which they have acquired a good title by 40 years' enjoyment'. They lost confidence, he wrote somewhat disingenuously, and were easily exploited and anxious and yet, occasionally, the menopause 'imparts a firmness of purpose' when a more 'masculine character' was assumed, and women were 'less subject to be led astray by a too ardent imagination, or by wild flights of passion'. Don't for a minute think this is good news because, as 'Time dulls the eye, robs the cheek of its bloom, delves furrows in the forehead [it] cannot quell the seraphic fire burning in the heart of women' and their residual femininity should 'prompt them to deeds of charity' rather than adventure. She had to be careful, given these restrictions, that she didn't allow herself to become 'peevish, harsh, dismal . . . viewing everything through a jaundiced veil', and should, of course, fully 'accept her new position'. Tilt did his level best to emphasize the 'many indispositions and diseases pertinacious, complicated, and shrouded in such misty confusion' which beset menopausal women and 'one by one snap the cords which anchor (a woman) to life. At 50 parents may have been gathered to the dust, children may have deserted the parental roof . . . doubts rise whether with faded charms . . . she can possibly retain possession of her husband's affection.'

You might be forgiven for thinking that all this advice was enough to send anybody mad, and indeed it probably did. Tilt, for one, placed enormous emphasis on nervous diseases, maintaining, in line with previous medical opinion, that the 'poor suffer less than the rich. Luxury is the hot-bed of nervous afflictions' – luxury being an enforced lack of meaningful occupation, hence the injunction to charitable works. The menopause could engender insanity, mania, hypochondriasis, melancholia, apathy, delirium, hysteria, pseudo-narcotism, chlorosis and syncope, to name a few. Tilt's observations drew on his detailed case histories: he diagnosed one Mary W. as displaying 'Melancholia, with suicidal tendencies, caused by cessation'. Mary was a 'tall athletic woman, with a pale face, iron-grey hair, a whimpering tone of voice, and apparently always ready to cry'. She was forty-five and the wife of a publican 'in good circumstances' when she came to the Farringdon Dispensary in November 1855. Tilt recorded that her 'm. flow appeared at 13, and came regularly . . . she had borne several children . . . but it ceased suddenly 8 months before I saw her'. He also noted that she was passing blood through her bowels, had a painful and enlarged abdomen and had been 'thought pregnant by a high obstetric authority'. For the 'last few months she suffered much from dry flushes during the day, and from "her skin stinging and perspiring" during the night. "All this", says the patient, "I could easily bear, were it not for my nervous state".' She complained of being 'all a tremble . . . sleepless all night, and powerless all day . . . she sits alone, doleful and disconsolate, ashamed of herself for being so lazy, and still unable to do anything, or forgetful of what it is she ought to do . . . she often despairs of Providence, and is much afflicted with suicidal thoughts'. Tilt prescribed his 'usual mixture before meals' of carbonated soda, 'blue pill', and hyoscyamus every other night, Dover's Powder every night, a large belladonna plaster at the pit of the stomach and vaginal injections with a solution of acetate of lead. Three months later, in February 1856, he had her on opium and by March she was 'in every way better', even though he described her motions as 'bloody'. By the next month she was telling him that her 'gloomy fits and suicidal tendencies' were improving, though this was accompanied by an 'increasing amount of flushes and perspirations' and she had 'grown suddenly stouter, although eating very little'. She refused to have three ounces of blood taken from her arm, despite pressure from Tilt, who 'told her she could not be cured without'. In May she passed blood from her vagina and bowels 'after a scene with her drunken husband'. Tilt now prescribed a mixture of hydrochlorate of morphine, chloric ether and distilled water to be taken by the tablespoonful, three times a day. By August she looked seven months' pregnant, was bilious, still passing bloody motions, 'but', wrote the apparently oblivious Tilt, 'her health and appearance have surprisingly improved, notwithstanding the worry of sick children, and a home ruined by the bankruptcy of an unkind husband'. He saw her for the last time nearly a year after she first came to him and wrote, tellingly, that 'she continued in good health, although she had left off the medicines'.

Another of his patients, a Mrs L, aged fifty-four, he described as melancholic. She was inclined to 'sit by the fire all day absorbed in transacting strange things with strange people of former times, and often frightened by ghastly faces'. She confided that she felt an 'uncontrollable impulse to move about, and to dash her head against the wall . . . then sinking down again, to remain immobile for hours'. Mrs L agreed to let Tilt bleed her, ten ounces from her arm; he gave her a purgative, a dose of morphine to be taken every night, and ordered regular, tepid, two-hour baths as if to physically dissolve her miseries. After four weeks of this regime she had several months of the proprietary medicine Dover's Powder, nightly, a 'composing' diaphoretic or sweat-inducing compound of ipecacuanha, opium and a cooling salt, perhaps sulphate of potassium. To top this off she was to apply a belladonna and opium plaster to the pit of her stomach, but it was a 'tour to the German spas with a valued friend [which] completed the cure'. One can't help but feel that it was the trip away with a woman friend and a break from the drugs and the purging that really made her feel better.

Some of Tilt's patients exhibited temper, a craving for spirits or 'oinomania', an impulse to steal, to murder, to attempt suicide, recklessness with money, fear of penury and the workhouse, 'demonomania' or a belief in Satanic influence – that the Devil had 'lodged in her womb', or had 'taken up his abode in each hipbone'. When menopausal women committed crimes Tilt chose to believe they were victims of their biology, arguing that if judges 'admit that parturition determines uncontrollable impulses, they must also allow the possible occurrence of the same impulse at all critical stages of a woman's life', including at cessation, when irrational creatures with no greater control than beasts might react wildly. While some physicians still adhered to the idea of 'hysterical delirium and convulsions' being attributable to the retention of poisonous blood that 'ought to have been eliminated by the menstrual flow', Tilt thought that the ovaries were acting on the brain through the nervous system rather than via the blood flow. 'Something', he wrote, was sent to the brain so that woman was 'no longer the mistress of her own actions, was literally "fuddled with animal spirits, and made giddy with constitutional joy"'. While 'involution is taking place, the ovaries disturb the viscera with which they have worked harmoniously for 30 years . . . I do not pretend to know the nature of this disturbing influence, but I suppose it is similar to that made manifest by the coming into power of the ovaries at puberty.' All was 'vague and hazardous' and he strove to bring order and exact knowledge with statistical analysis. In this he both reflected ancient thinking and prefigured the ideas of the late-nineteenth-century endocrinologists.

One author writing on Tilt in the 1980s thought that he 'was ideally suited to be a gynaecologist' being a 'very tall, handsome man, erect and spare in figure, very particular in his dress and courteous in his manner . . . much esteemed by those who consulted him'. He had a large practice drawn from 'the upper classes of society' and many American women crossed the Atlantic to see him. This is all pretty alarming, seeming as it does to sexualize and romanticize the male gynaecologist who, with seductive airs, would patronize and overwhelm his patients with his suave good looks. It says much about ideas on the menopause in the late twentieth century, let alone Tilt's in the mid nineteenth.

In the quarter of a century after Tilt's works were first published 'the whole pathology of gynaecology [was] so modified that it [became] virtually new'.[30] This at least was A. D. Leith Napier's claim for his book *The Menopause and its Disorders* (1897), and he did attempt a greater objectivity about his subject, putting it in historical context. Napier went back to examine and compare ancient and contemporary theories of menstruation, understanding that it was necessary to study menstruation in order to understand menopause. He thought some theories just plain wrong, founded on a rudimentary, incomplete knowledge of heredity and the process of civilization. The idea that menstruation is but one consequence of women's different 'sentiments' and the 'restraint of their sexual instinct' was nonsense, he thought, arguing that apes also menstruated but did not wear bustles or take tea. The ovulation theory of menstruation did not hold water for him either, as modern research suggested that ovulation could occur without menstruation and could take place before puberty and even, apparently, after the menopause. Concluding that no theory could be satisfactorily demonstrated, Napier bravely proposed that much of medicine's knowledge was based on assumptions and so much guesswork. 'It is not easy,' he wrote, 'to precisely define what is to be regarded as normal in relation to the menopause.'

What was needed was a '*reliable* account of subjective symptoms or sensations from a very large number of seemingly healthy women' and to make a series of examinations of them. 'Obviously women only consult a medical practitioner when they have, or believe they have, some definite reason for doing so', and this meant that the influence of menopause had been exaggerated and 'many evils' had been attributed to it 'which investigation proves to be only co-existent'. On the other hand, there was 'no doubt that the term "c. of l." has been, nay, still is . . . employed as a convenient cloak for hiding the laziness of the physician, or as a vague description . . . for allaying anxieties'. It is a 'great transitional epoch in the woman's existence' and 'must be distinguished from the properly senile even though the menopause is the beginning of old age and devolution'.[31]

The homeopath James Compton Burnett also exhorted his colleagues to listen attentively and sympathetically to the 'health-histories of a few score ladies in their sufferings at the change of life'. He believed that an 'absolutely healthy woman changes without any ills whatever', and a 'normal woman, married or maiden, who has no disease or disease taint, has nothing to fear from the change of life'. But why, he asked, disingenuously, 'do we think and speak of the change of life almost as if it were of necessity a dangerous, mysterious period that all women should and do dread?' Because, and here's the catch, 'few are truly free from disease and taintless'; moreover, these few 'do not throng our consulting-rooms [and] a medical man is hardly a fair judge of the number of really normal persons, for the very sufficient reason that such individuals need no physician, and rarely come to him'. The errors that orthodox medics made in recommending certain treatments were 'damnable'; douches, for example, were 'nasty and vulgar to boot . . . in fact a dirty proceeding'. He complained that he had never heard a clinical lecture, or read an article or book on the menopause that was the least help to him in his practice. The menopause was, 'to say the least, a very dark region indeed wherein we are left to grope about in quest of unknown quasi-ghostlike awfulnesses'. Like the explorers Burton and Speke he had 'tried at least to strike a match in any dark corner' where 'mysteries midst ghostly terrors abound; and although the illumination emanating from one solitary match is not exactly blinding, still it is more helpful than utter darkness'. The 'evil repute of the change of life in women' led inexorably to their resignation to suffering, and he found it 'absolutely astonishing' that they submitted so easily. His enlightened approach stretched only so far, however, because he assured his peers that the 'troubles at the change of life . . . date from, often, far back in their lives, or in the lives of their parents'. These troubles were in fact 'nature's wreakings of wrathful vengeance for persistent dis-obedience'. In the rare 'normal' woman periods cease as they began, 'almost imperceptibly: it just leaves off, and there is an end to it', but for women whose menopause was 'looming', who had lived more chaotic lives and whose wombs were 'fagged', the pre-existent taint once carried off by menstrual blood was deposited in the body and could cause cancers.

Knowledge about the menstrual cycle was extremely poor and only relatively recently has it begun to be better understood. It wasn't until 1930 that there was conclusive proof that ovulation occurs midway between two periods, a fact observed by a Japanese gynaecologist, Kaysaku Ogino, who laparotomized women at various stages of their cycle. Previously, a French anatomist, Professor Pouchet of Rouen, had maintained in his *Ten Fundamental Laws of Reproduction* (1842) that a woman ovulated at menstruation, and had advocated a disastrous rhythm method of contraception based on this mistake. The following year another physician, Professor Raciborski in Paris, argued that as he had known women to conceive without bleeding when they had married immediately after a period, they could not possibly be ovulating at menstruation. Women who married later in their cycles almost invariably menstruated again before they conceived.[32]

In the nineteenth century most physicians still followed the Greek idea of menstruation as a purging or cleansing, a physiological bloodletting, and in cases where menstruation was suppressed it was thought that other organs would produce vicarious periodic haemorrhages from the nose, anus, gums, kidneys or nipples. Men, too, might menstruate under this theory: an obstetrician, Alfred Wiltshire, writing on male 'menstruation' in the *Lancet* in 1885, reported the case of a surgeon who bled from his penis every three weeks, and an American physician recorded that of a medical student who had had 'an apparent catamenial secretion, with the same regularity' for three years, 'attended by the same indications by which it is characterised in the human female'. But men could not ovulate, and by 1850 the 'ovular theory' of menstruation was being used to explain the biological basis of femininity, the ovaries having been established as the 'grand organs' of sexual activity and difference, encompassing 'the drive that most firmly binds man to the animal level'. Ovaries defined women and inextricably bound them to animality: they were primitive and struggled for reason and intellect.[33] Perfectly illustrating this supposition, James MacGrigor Allan, addressing the Anthropological Society in London in 1869, informed his audience that menstruating 'women are unfit for any great mental or physical labour'. Moreover, they 'suffer under a languor and depression which disqualify them for thought or action, and render it extremely doubtful how they can be considered responsible beings while the crisis lasts'. Knowing, as he most surely thought he did, the true nature of 'normal' femininity, Allan understood how insanity was closely linked to the mysterious workings of the ovaries. 'It is not improbable,' he continued, 'that instances of feminine cruelty (which startle us as so inconsistent with the normal gentleness of the sex) are attributable to mental excitement caused by their periodic illness.' Along with Michelet, who defined woman as an invalid and 'eternally wounded' to boot, Allan agreed that:

> Such she emphatically is, as compared with man . . . In intellectual labour, man has surpassed, does now, and always will surpass woman, for the obvious reason that nature does not periodically interrupt his thought and application.[34]

To the medical profession woman was her biological self and no more, and from this cruelly simplistic 'fact' flowed assumptions of femininity, virtue, morality and wider social ideas about who and what she was or might be. There was no parallel scientific study of masculinity or andrology, an omission that reflected the ancient belief of an ideal male body and an imperfect, problematic female one.[35] Braxton Hicks, lecturing in 1877 on the difference between the sexes, did allow that the terms 'climacteric' and 'turn of life' could also be applied to men ('menopause' being applicable only to women), though 'in him the change is more gradual'.[36] He thought it a neutral, man-woman state in which she was 'less of the woman she was than a man is a man at the same time of life'. Alexander Skene, in *Medical Gynaecology: A Treatise on the Diseases of Women from the Standpoint of the Physician* (1895), called it the 'death of the woman in the woman', whilst G. Delauney, on 'Equality and inequality in sex' in *Popular Science Monthly* 20 (December 1881), had cited 'intellectual and moral differences' to explain why,

> in higher societies, the two sexes . . . become separated during the age of maturity, and become again more alike in old age . . . at about forty-five years the distinctions begin to attenuate, and the sexes end by resembling each other . . . when the characteristics are rather masculine.[37]

The difference, and so the opposition, of the sexes was validated by scientific fact. Gynaecology, according to the *New Universal Etymological, Technological, and Pronouncing Dictionary of the English Language* (1849), was the 'doctrine of the nature and diseases of women'. By 'women' they meant reproductive organs, no more, no less.[38] The acceptance of woman's difference and her subordination to her reproductive function was constantly reiterated and emphasized in medical texts. William Tyler Smith made it plain in the *Lancet* in 1848 that women 'stood at the boundary between physiology and pathology'. Professor M. L. Holbrook, speaking to fellow medics in 1870, assured them that 'the Almighty, in creating

the female sex, had taken the uterus and built up a woman
around it'. Robert Barnes, writing in the 1882 edition of
Quain's *Dictionary of Medicine* on the scope of gynaecology,
stated, without going so far as to actually agree that 'the life
of woman is a history of disease', that

> it is undeniable that to appreciate justly the pathology of
> women we must observe her in all her social relations, study
> minutely her moral and intellectual characteristics – that
> we must in short, never for a moment lose sight of those
> physical attributes which indelibly stamp her as a woman,
> which direct, control, and limit the exercise of her faculties.
> This collateral study is of infinitely more importance in the
> pathological history of woman than it is of man.

The pathology of the male sexual system has never been seen
to define men's nature in the way that a woman's has hers.
Barnes wrote a *Clinical History of the Medical and Surgical Diseases of
Women* (1882) and baldly stated that 'Any disease occurring in a
woman will almost certainly involve some modifications in
the work of her sexual system.' And even the 'ordinary or disturbed work of her sexual system will influence the course of
any disease which may assail her, however independent this
disease may seem in its origin.'[39] In the *Lancet* in 1873 he wrote
that her 'climacteric perturbation is often even more marked
than what is observed at any previous period of life . . . It is a
stage of transition and of trial for all . . . many women have
passed through the trials of puberty and child bearing without
serious nervous disorder and will break down at menopause.'[40]

The ovaries were the seat of feminine essence and all that
was virtuous in Victorian woman sprang from their operation, but if they were diseased, if she behaved in a less than

passive and ladylike manner, then all hell could break loose. W. W. Bliss, in his work *Woman and Her Thirty-Years' Pilgrimage* (Boston, 1870), propagated 'these views of the gigantic power and influence of the ovaries over the whole animal economy of woman . . . they are the most powerful agents in all the commotions of her system'. These innocent organs predicted her intellect, her standing in society, her physical perfection, and

> all that lends beauty to those fine and delicate contours which are constant objects of admiration, all that is great, noble and beautiful, all that is voluptuous, tender, and endearing; that her fidelity, her devotedness, her perpetual vigilance, forecast, and all those qualities of mind and disposition that inspire respect and love and fit her as the safest counsellor and friend of man.

Imagine, then, if she is in fact the sum of her ovaries alone *'what must be their influence and power over the great vocation of woman and the august purposes of her existence when these organs have become compromised through disease!'*[41] But, hellish problem: 'extirpation of the ovaries' could cause a woman to 'become thinner, and more apparently muscular; her breasts, which were large, are gone' and, of course, she would cease to menstruate, attracting all manner of new dangers, including the perversion of her sexual feelings.[42] Perhaps women could be greatly improved by having their troublesome ovaries cut out; they would be more biddable, orderly, industrious and so much cleaner in mind and body, their moral status enhanced. The influence of 'diseased' ovaries could be disastrous for the woman, her husband, family and society at large, for the negative effect of the organs on her mind contained all 'artfulness and dissimulation'. An ovariotomy might be in order if she displayed a hearty appetite, masturbated or showed any erotic interest, attempted suicide, revealed 'cussedness', had dysmenorrhea or, unsurprisingly, a persecution mania. Better to have them out, better to have her spayed, as the surgeon John Hunter had suggested in the eighteenth century.

Medical knowledge was not an autonomous system of thought: social, cultural, political and commercial spheres influenced the direction and choice of physicians in diseases and therapies. The choices they made and the routes they followed transformed perceptions of the human body. They had significant bearing on the way society organized itself and how individuals saw themselves in relation to each other during the nineteenth century.[43] Medicine was politics and economics as well as knowledge and craft, and the menopause became a lucrative niche open to new exploration and, inevitably, exploitation. The contradictory, the messy and the anecdotal were crystallized into scientific theory, giving an impression of validity and consensus. Based on limited, largely male, experience and an accumulation of medical knowledge and prejudice, the menopause was stitched together in patchwork fashion. But though the scientific understanding of physiology had grown and treatments become more sophisticated – and some arguably more dangerous – little else had changed in the last 200 years.

5

KNIVES AND ASYLUMS

Wonderful, indeed, is woman's hydra-like tolerance of sections
and mutilations under their hands.

Sir Spencer Wells (1891)

'Gynaecology,' wrote Tilt in his *Handbook of Uterine Therapeutics*
(1863), 'or the accurate study of diseases of women, is the
youngest branch of medical literature, for it began in 1816.' A
veritable 'galaxy of Paris physicians' had brought the 'sexual
organs of women within the range of the general law of
pathology'. From the beginning of the nineteenth century,
despite some physicians' opposition to surgical recklessness,
there were a few who began to perform gynaecological procedures on women, sometimes for dubious and often
unspecified reasons. Many of these operations caused premature menopause with devastating consequences for the
future lives of the women concerned. The scientific and professional credibility of surgery was on the increase and many
of the operations were daringly innovative, if potentially

terribly dangerous.[1] This was especially the case in America, where the medical profession was less regulated, particularly in the southern states where there was a ready supply of slaves to experiment and practise upon.[2] Tilt praised the French for their elegant journey to the final frontier of women's bodies but damned the 'intrusion of surgical Americanism' and their 'operative debauchery', saying, 'now, in America, the womb is to have no peace'.

As with any major internal surgery, surgical gynaecology became popular only with the advent of anaesthesia and anti-septic procedures. The writer and diarist Fanny Burney's account of the mastectomy she underwent without anaes-thetic in 1811 at the age of fifty-nine gives a frighteningly clear idea of what this meant. After discovering a lump in her breast she initially tried a long dietary regimen but, when the painful lump was the size of her fist and made her full of 'dread repugnance', she finally consulted Napoleon's cele-brated army-surgeon, Dominique-Jean Larrey. He did not see her breast until the day of the operation and even then did not touch her during his examination. She wrote:

Everything convinced me . . . that this experiment alone could save me . . . I mounted, therefore, unbidden, the Bed stead – & M. Dubois placed upon me the mattress, & spread a cambric handkerchief upon my face. It was transparent, however, & I saw, through it, that the Bed stead was instantly surrounded by the 7 men & my nurse. I refused to be held; but when, Bright through the cambric, I saw the glitter of polished Steel – I closed my Eyes. I would not trust to con-vulsive fear the sight of the terrible incision . . . a terror that surpasses all description, & the most torturing pain. Yet – when the dreadful steel was plunged into the breast –

cutting through veins – arteries – flesh – nerves – I needed
no injunctions not to restrain my cries. I began a scream that
lasted unintermittingly during the whole time of the incision – & I almost marvel that it rings not in my Ears still! So
excruciating was the agony. When the wound was made, &
the instrument was withdrawn, the pain seemed undimin-
ished, for the air that suddenly rushed into those delicate
parts felt like a mass of minute but sharp & forked poniards,
that were tearing the edges of the wound – but when again
I felt the instrument – describing a curve – cutting against
the grain . . . while the flesh resisted in a manner so forcible
as to oppose & tire the hand of the operator, who was forced
to change from the right to the left – then, indeed, I thought
I must have expired. I attempted no more to open my Eyes, –
they felt as if hermetically shut, & so firmly closed, that the
Eyelids seemed indented into the Cheeks.

She felt 'the Knife rackling against the breast bone – scraping
it!' and even, with a terrible sensitivity, the doctor's hand above
her, 'though I saw nothing, & though he touched nothing'.
Afterwards her strength was 'totally annihilated'. It has been
suggested, given that she lived for another twenty-nine years,
that the lump had been benign and the operation unnecessary. Without Larrey's surgical speed and expertise, perfected
on the battlefields where many surgeons had polished their
skills, Burney may not have survived the appalling ordeal.[3]

Jane Todd Crawford, a 47-year-old widow, had her ovaries
cut out in 1809 without anaesthesia and before physicians
had any knowledge of how to prevent infection. Her physician, Ephraim McDowell from Kentucky, had studied in
Edinburgh under John Bell, the influential anatomist and
surgeon, and had returned to America to practise.

Astonishingly, Jane not only survived but lived on for another thirty-one years. Another American, the prolific John Attlee, removed the ovaries of seventy-eight women between 1843 and 1883, sixty-four of whom recovered. But mortality rates were extremely high, running at about 50 per cent, and this would improve only with the introduction of antisepsis, asepsis, general anaesthesia, blood transfusion and antibiotics, and these fully benefited women only in about the middle of the twentieth century.

In mid-nineteenth-century Alabama James Marion Sims, who has been called the 'father figure of gynaecology', was operating extensively on black female slaves – one of whom underwent surgery thirty times in four years.[4] Later in a New York hospital he refined his technique, using the poorest of Irish immigrant women. By 1906 it was estimated that at least 150,000 women in America had had the newly fashionable ovariotomy, and some of these operations had been performed by women: Mary Dixon Jones, despite warning against over-aggressive surgery, performed countless ovariotomies. Her alleged 'lack of female empathy' was blamed for her professional demise, but the necessity of working within a male-dominated profession on females must surely have produced a great deal of conflict. Women physicians had a personal interest in the definitions and treatments of their own sex, not least because many (male) gynaecologists argued that, being female, they were quite unfit to practise medicine. These women often saw themselves as proof that their sex should not be dismissed by the reductive idea of woman-as-womb.[5]

The first French woman to be licensed as a physician and pharmacist, Hélina Gaboriau, denounced gynaecological surgery in her pragmatically titled work *Normal Feminine Medicine*, of the early 1900s, though it has to be said she was busy pushing her husband's tonics and unguents as the alternative treatment. Influential figures such as Victor Hugo and Emile Zola supported the movement to 'protect women against surgical abuse'. There were suspicions of ovariotomies being used as a contraceptive or abortive procedure and Zola's novel *Fécondité* (1899) contained a storyline of this nature. The book was considered by the medical profession to be well researched. The heroine, Sérafine, has her ovaries removed and is glad to be rid of the fear of pregnancy but, in line with medical thought, she loses her sexual desire, her femininity and her youthfulness.

In Britain, ovariotomy was first performed in 1824 by an Edinburgh surgeon and lecturer in anatomy and physiology, John Lizars, and though this patient survived, his next three did not.[6] By mid-century over 130 such operations had been carried out, and by 1855, out of 200 operations, the mortality rate stood at 44.5 per cent. Sir Spencer Wells, in London, was operating on a regular basis and managed to reduce mortality from more than 50 per cent to 11 per cent over the next two decades, largely due to the introduction of anaesthesia in the late 1840s. He maintained that he performed this surgery to relieve the suffering of women, but some of his colleagues, including the eminent Professor Robert Lee, who spoke at a meeting of the Royal Medico-Chirurgical Society in Scotland in 1862, believed the benefits were to the surgeons alone, in their financial and professional gains.[7] Lee was no small-time opponent but a prolific and influential if conservative physician, working on the anatomical structure and development of the nerves of the uterus and heart, midwifery, hysteria, puerperal inflammation, tubal gestation and ovarian cysts, sterility, premature labour and the use of the speculum. According to Lee's obituary in the *BMJ* in March 1877, he was so sure that his 'convictions were the results of hard and well-intentioned study; so sure that he sought the truth, and sought it in the right way, that he was wholly unable to believe that any one, with equal honesty, and almost equal industry' could arrive at different conclusions. Another British surgeon, Robert Liston, condemned the ovariotomists as 'belly rippers', whilst some suggested the operations were nothing better than vivisection carried out for the sake of scientific curiosity and surgical practice.[8]

Wells did object to the oöphorectomy, a 'normal ovariotomy' as it was known in America, or Battey's operation, after the surgeon Robert Battey working in the 1870s, where ovaries were removed to alleviate menstrual problems but with no real indication as to whether the organs were diseased or not. Protesting too much perhaps, or stung by the criticism his own practice had received, Wells accused those who performed oöphorectomy of being uncivilized, unscrupulous and 'illogically enthusiastic experimenters'. An oöphorectomy carried out by Francis Imlach on a Mrs Casey in Liverpool in 1886 divided the profession and outraged the public even more. Imlach found himself in a court of law charged with removing her ovaries and Fallopian tubes without any proven necessity and without her consent. Mrs Casey herself testified that she had experienced menopause as a result of the operation, which had precipitated 'a change not only in her own life, but in the life of her husband'. Imlach was found not guilty but nevertheless lost his gynaecological practice. Inpatients at the hospital that year had numbered just 347, and the statement that 111 of these, nearly one third, had undergone abdominal section caused almost universal horror amid claims that the women of Liverpool were being unsexed and experimented on.[9] Some argued that the operation did not eliminate sexual desire because that feeling resided in the nervous system and not the ovaries. Sherwood-Dunn, a gynaecologist writing in the *Transactions of the American Association of Obstetricians and Gynaecologists*, reported that, out of more than 400 cases he had tabulated, not one had experienced a total loss of sexual feeling, and only three women had noticed any marked diminution in 'the sexual feeling' after a period of three years following the operation.[10]

According to J. B. Hicks in a piece submitted to the *BMJ* in 1877, 'On the difference between the sexes in regard to the aspect and treatment of disease', loss of feelings of arousal, a reversion to 'the neutral man-woman state', might make a woman 'more capable of rendering herself useful . . . free from sexual activity and its many demands on the powers of the system at this later period of life'. She would suffer less from disease and be 'more secure against external battles and exposure to the elements; more cared for, she more frequently outlives her male comrade in the battle for life'.[11] But Rudolf Virchow, physician, anthropologist, public health campaigner and politician, warned that to 'remove the ovary [means] we shall have before us a masculine woman . . . ugly half-form with the coarse and harsh features, the heavy bone formation, the moustache, the rough voice, the flat chest, the sour and egotistic mentality and the distorted outlook'. Virchow seems to display a touch of indirect male self-loathing here, or a disgust with woman 'not fit for purpose'. In short, he writes, 'all that we admire and respect in woman as womanly, is merely dependent on her ovaries'.[12] Without these organs, or without their functioning, a woman is no longer a real woman, but neither is she admired for her acquired 'masculine' qualities. She is diseased or deranged, or has just disappeared.

A dire lack of consensus and understanding wrapped in opinion was standing in for observation, experience and a priori scientific evidence. As gynaecologists tried to consolidate and protect their professional status and knowledge, and to develop 'safer', anaesthetized surgical skills, they were manipulating femaleness and female sexuality to fit their own needs, both selfish and altruistic. Gregorio Marañón's vision of gynaecology acknowledged the 'danger in confusing hypotheses with evident truths', but he himself was reduced to using fictional examples to illustrate his ideas, faced as he and his profession still were with so little real knowledge. He defended the use of fiction with the curious claim that 'excessive contact with the material blunts [a physician's] psychologic penetration', a 'phenomenon . . . especially patent among gynaecologists'. Indeed, 'contrary to what excitable adolescents believe', a woman's genitals were her 'least intimate' parts.[13] Quoting the heroine of Michaelis's 'admirable' novel *L'Âge Dangereux* (1911), he continued, 'I have spoken with many famous gynaecologists and I have admired their knowledge. But in my heart I laugh at their simplicity. They know how to cut open and sew up, like children with their dolls. But they go no further than that.' Here lies the rub. Marañón and his peers (unlike Tilt and his more grandiose, philosophic claims) lacked the ability to see 'what lies behind in the privacy of the human soul, inaccessible to the professional eye, medical or clerical'.[14] But it didn't stop them trying.

Marañón's work echoed Tilt's of over seventy years before, and he agreed with his predecessor that doctors would still have a 'hard time finding a comprehensive and modern study of the climacteric tradition'. There was, he complained, 'more literature on almost any rare disease, which will, perhaps, not be presented more than once in a whole lifetime of medical practice, than a menopausal physiopathology'. This neglect presented Marañón with the opportunity to fill the void with his deeply detailed study of the problematic and 'curious fact' of the menopause. Proud believers in the progress of medical science were thrilled that female genitalia were no longer viewed as some sort of sentimentally venerated monstrance. James Murphy, addressing the first Congress of the British Gynaecological Society in 1891, had told his assembled colleagues that at the beginning of the century

> the female genital organs were regarded as so mysterious and so sacred that no matter how serious the disease that afflicted them might be, it was no justification for an examination either by sight or by touch, and as long as that state of affairs continued there naturally was no work for the hand of the surgeon.

In language awash with sexual metaphor and the triumph of male gaze and action, he praised the 'modern gynaecologist' who 'has shorn the female genitalia of their mystery, and examined by sight and touch every portion of them, and has successfully attacked their disease with scalpel and scissors'. It is little wonder that practitioners were accused by some of 'castration' and of 'instrumental rape'.

The ideological position of women in society was reiterated in medical language, and the medical right to penetrate and violate – and the anxiety about taking this right – lay just below the surface of a sometimes quite hysterical speculum controversy. Hippocrates was said to have used a variation of the speculum, but Soranus of Ephesus is the first author who mentions the vaginal speculum, a tube introduced into the vagina so that the cervix could be directly inspected. The *dioptra* was one of the most spectacular Graeco-Roman medical instruments, superior in its precision and smooth phallic shape to the later European Renaissance *priapiscus*. Three bronze examples were dug from the ruins of Pompeii in 1818, made up of three branches, two handles and a screw in the centre. The instrument was reintroduced in 1801 by Joseph Récamier, Professor of Medicine at the Collège de France in Paris. Within a decade, Parisian authorities had sanctioned its 'barbarous' use on suspected prostitutes under the sanitary laws so that it became an instrument of the police. Women could now be internally examined in the presence of public witnesses, 'although lighting the dark depths was a problem'. In a startling display of the double-standard, the police used it on prostitutes, to separate the clean from the unclean and to prevent partly cured women being 'turned out "well", merely to infect fresh men'. Men, by implication, were not considered carriers of disease. British and American medical students in Paris took the instrument, and its terrible new reputation, home with them.[15] In Britain the controversial Contagious Diseases Acts of 1864 and 1866, designed to 'Prevent the Spreading of Contagious Diseases' and 'make vice safe for men', made the speculum an instrument of the British police, too, allowing them and JPs, inspectors, magistrates and medical practitioners to apprehend any woman they suspected of prostitution, detain and examine her against her will and without her consent. If she refused she faced a prison sentence. The French, however, were proud of the speculum and fiercely debated the practice of ovariotomies and hysterectomies, believing that their tradition of gynaecological examination ruled out the need for such invasive surgery. Internal examination of women, with the doctor's fingers introduced into the vagina, was fraught with real and imaginary worries, especially in Anglo-Saxon countries. 'Matters', though, 'were somewhat different with the Latins', where an expected female modesty and male sensibility struggled with fears of an immoderate or unwholesome interest or misplaced sexual desire.[16]

By 1849 a piece in the *London Journal of Medicine* on 'Digital Examination, and the Speculum: Their Uses and Abuses' highlighted a growing 'feeling against an indiscriminate but too common reliance on the Speculum [which] seems to be gaining strength both in this country and in France'. The author, William Acton, could only hope that 'while the evils and improprieties connected with the abuse of this instrument are exposed and denounced, the current of professional opinion may not set in too strongly against its employment'. Acton argued too that drugs and washes had been abused in the treatment of female diseases but hardly anyone was against their use. William Tyler Smith was one who did have a moral objection to the administration of these anaesthetic agents, one which 'should unite against them all men who desire to hold up the respectability of the obstetric department of medicine; for most assuredly, the present kind of attendance could not continue if the facts were understood by parents and husbands': those in charge of women whose sexually uninhibited self often emerged under the influence of the drugs. A case of control producing an opposite and very undesirable effect to the supine one required. And George Gregory wondered 'how much affection is left for the poor husband?' after his wife had been through such an experience.[17]

Robert Lee, speaking before the Royal Medical and

Chirurgical Society in London in 1850, seriously doubted the 'legitimate and real value' of the speculum, detailing abuses and insisting that it was completely 'unjustifiable on the grounds of propriety and morality'. Lee attacked the 'apostles of the speculum', citing the case of a middle-aged woman with paraplegia whose physician, believing her symptoms arose from her uterus even though she had never suffered from any gynaecological disease, insisted on using the speculum to examine her. A second physician present was shocked by what happened, relating that all the doors had to be closed to prevent her screams being heard. The following week she died of an inflammation at the base of her brain; her uterus had been quite healthy.[18] In 1857 the Royal Medical and Chirurgical Society let it be known that it would have been better for the pure women of England had the speculum remained confined to the foul French syphilitic wards, no instrument being more subversive of female delicacy and more capable of ready abuse.

Thomas Litchfield condemned the 'filthy and indecent application' of the speculum, picturing in vivid terms 'the terror depicted in [a] poor lady's countenance when such was proposed by the doctor, and she ran behind me, exclaiming, with apparent horror, to save her from such an infliction, and exclaiming, "No, no! let me alone; I will die as I am."' The Lancet doubted whether patients would 'submit' to the speculum when physicians themselves obviously considered it indecent. And the effect on the women physically, but more especially morally, could be, according to some, quite catastrophic. Robert Brudenell Carter, in his work On the Pathology and Treatment of Hysteria (London, 1853), said that he had known women 'of the middle classes of society, reduced, by the constant use of the speculum, to the mental and moral condition of prostitutes; seeking to give themselves the same indulgence by the practice of solitary vice; and asking every medical practitioner, under whose care they fell, to institute an examination of the sexual organs'. The danger of corrupting the patient went hand in hand with the potential corruption of the medical practitioner who could metamorphose in a Jekyll and Hyde manner into 'a man who is moved by sinister motives, dishonest, and extortionate, who makes a trade of his profession'. A Dr Parrish elaborated on the gothic scenario in 1854, imagining a physician cajoling his vulnerable menopausal patient with the words:

> You are approaching the critical time of life. Your womb is extremely irritable; it is very feeble, and you are liable to sudden and dangerous hemorrhage. If you do not allow me to prescribe for you regularly till you pass this *fearful* crisis, I cannot be responsible for the issue. All this clotted blood probably comes from some organic change . . . It may be the commencement of a cancer . . .

He then arranges an appointment with her and

> the speculum and the dreaded case of instruments, with all the paraphernalia incident to this species of quackery are displayed. The womb is exposed to view. Females, who have never before seen the organ, are now quietly indulged with a sight, and erudite explanations whispered into their ears, and then their testimony secured to sustain the opinion of the *animal* who conducts the examination . . . In the course of nature the [menstrual] discharge soon ceases. The patient is free from her apprehensions, and goes from

neighbour to neighbour, to laud the skill of the being who has miraculously saved her from death; while he appropriates a large fee.[19]

Sensational pieces in medical journals suggested 'crowds of women rushed to a gentleman's door, begging to have the speculum used [with] abandoned eagerness'. Many doctors believed the instrument was a real threat to the happiness of family life as women all succumbed to this 'new and lamentable form of hysteria'. It was thought so potentially corrupting that a woman's mind, particularly if she was unmarried, could be irretrievably poisoned by the experience. She was certainly no longer 'the same person in delicacy and purity that she was before', indeed the physician should be wary of his patient as a seductress who would try and tempt him into inserting his speculum for her unnatural sexual gratification. She might develop moodiness, perversion and introspection, and even be so dreadfully affected that she would begin to speak unintelligibly, stuttering in broken sentences. Women, everybody knew, were of a highly nervous temperament and it followed that 'exciting modes of treatment must be avoided' lest the attentions of a speculum-wielding physician should become preferable to those of a lawful conjugal partner. Dr Heywood Smith knew that for women, 'when they are touched and excited, a time arrived when, though not intending to sin, they lost all physical control over themselves'. Added to that was the influence of the aristocracy, the celebrities of their day, who, by common agreement and deference, always took the lead in new health fads. They could be held to blame: one had only to imagine the 'complicated misery for a husband should his wife be set upon by a titled advocate of this uterine quackery'.[20]

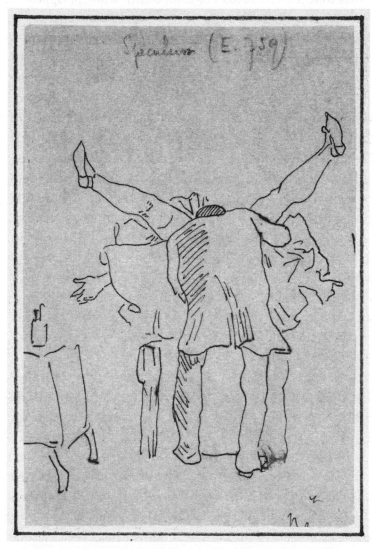

A Victorian gynaecologist wields his speculum to great effect.

Pro-specula physicians believed that there was 'no more harm in the use of the speculum than in the use of a spoon to ascertain the condition of the throat', as long as it was used by men of the highest integrity and not 'as a mere plaything to serve their own ends'. Radically, they argued that purity was in the mind, and could not be destroyed by the speculum. But others accused them of 'filthy and indecent application', mainly, it has to be said, through fear of losing the custom and 'the fast hold their noble science had on the middle and thoughtful classes'.

Increasingly, the debate began to centre on the efficacy of the kinds of specula available. The best of them, 'that of four blades', was deemed to be Madame Boivin's. Some were made of vulcanite with movable glass reflectors inside; others of opalescent glass, delicately and smoothly bevelled at each end. De la Bastie's deluxe toughened glass speculum was said to be less liable to shatter – unfortunately, many were known to 'explode suddenly and without any apparent cause'. The medical profession understood that 'should this occur during their introduction, or while *in situ* it would be extremely awkward'.[21] Tilt, in one of his many publications in the 1850s on the diseases of women, opined that the glass speculum was the most used in Britain:

> its diameter varies from half an inch to two inches, and the smoothness of its external coat of india-rubber, its high reflecting power, and the simplicity of its action, commend it to the beginner; it is the best for the application of leeches, or of a strong caustic . . . I have never found a glass speculum break in the vagina . . . but this accident did occur to a friend of mine in the country . . . the patient was very much frightened, and had to remain without

moving for several hours, while the doctor went for instruments and assistance.

Tilt thought that, though the speculum was 'inferior in value to the digital', it 'vastly improved the diagnoses of diseases of the womb, permitted some of them to be speedily and effectively cured, and gave to the study of diseases of women, an impetus that has already lasted fifty years, without showing signs of exhaustion'. At last, he thought, 'prejudice has given way to reason, and the speculum is now in general use, and by none more used than by those who first opposed it'. It was patently obvious, he wrote, that to make any kind of thorough specular examination, the clothes must be raised, but before doing so, 'each lower limb should be covered with a large cloth or thin shawl, if the patient does not wear drawers, for no part of the body should be uncovered, except that requiring investigation'.[22] Tilt's enthusiastic advocacy of the speculum followed him throughout his career and even made appearances in his obituaries, such was the intensity of feeling and opinion surrounding it.

Even with improved methods of diagnosis, no one was really sure how removing ovaries helped women suffering from uterine problems and, of course, mistakes were made in carrying out new surgical procedures. The 'flamboyant provincial gynaecologist' Lawson Tait admitted that 'our knowledge is incomplete and sometimes inaccurate' and that there were a 'few rare cases on record' where women had been injured by the use of obstetric implements in the hands of drunks or charlatans, 'unskilled operators' and those whose 'skill has been undone by intemperance', though not by any of his esteemed colleagues. Still, he himself had dealt with a case that resulted in the death of a woman and,

Strange to say, at the trial, a long array of skilled witnesses appeared for the defence, some of whom were hardy enough to declare that the procedure was a proper one under the circumstances, and that if they wrote books they would not hesitate to recommend it. The conviction and sentence which followed showed that the judge and jury were of a different opinion.[23]

Even towards the very end of the century when such surgery was pretty well established, there was a culture of silence and suppression protecting individual careers, the profession and medical innovation. In the *Journal of the American Medical Association* in 1899, J. E. Stubbs addressed his colleagues emphatically:

I warn all of you not to uncover the mistakes of a fellow practitioner because, if you do, it will come back like a boomerang . . . there are many cases that require extreme surgical dexterity and a large amount of knowledge in order to operate successfully; yet those who are operating all the time make mistakes. We have to do a great many things empirically, and if we tell people . . . this or that physician has made a great blunder, it hurts him; it hurts the community.[24]

By the end of the nineteenth century when surgical gynaecology was largely established, it was known that removal of the ovaries would result in cessation of menstruation. Marie Stopes, in her book *The Change of Life in Men and Women* (1936), railed against the fashion of 'twenty or more years ago [for] the medical profession to extirpate women's ovaries. For whatever reason this was done it had certain diabolical results.'[25] When both ovaries were removed by, as she put it, the criminally ignorant medicals of the day, women's femininity was destroyed in one attack on her most vital organs and an artificial menopause occurred which could produce a tendency towards masculinity, a deeper voice and facial hair. Millions of pounds had changed hands, Stopes reported angrily, and it had gone into the pockets of quacks and commercial beauty parlours because, naturally enough, women dislike the straggly coarse hair sometimes appearing at and after the menopause. Stopes advised plucking but, to back this up, 'a little ovarian extract combined with a little thyroid . . . will tend to keep the feminine balance'.

Ovariotomy was a fairly simple operation so it was used excessively in attempts to cure mental disorder, especially hysteria and nymphomania, which described the potential madness that could afflict a woman in times of crisis and cause her to be overwhelmed by sexual desire. The term 'hysteria' comes from the Greek, *hysterus*, meaning womb, and in the 1850s Tilt had called it 'the keystone of mental pathology'. The celebrated Parisian neurologist Jean-Martin Charcot defined it as the 'Great Neurosis' during the 1870s, and assured Freud in 1888 that 'hysteria is coming along, and one day it will occupy gloriously the important place it deserves in the sun'.[26] It was speculative then and is redundant now, a blanket metaphor for any suspicion of deviant female behaviour, especially of the sexual sort. Some menopausal women came to physicians suffering from 'pent-up sexual longings' which were, they said, much worse than mere pain: 'no sooner does night come on than I am prey to such dreadfully sinful desires that drive me mad'. Women's desires were generally seen as deriving from the maternal impulse alone, so when they were purely sexual they revealed an altogether more terrifying force as far as individuals and society were concerned. Thought irrational and more vulnerable to sexual disease, women were especially at risk of this particular physical and moral drain during critical periods of their lives, such as menopause.[27]

Samuel Ashwell thought it was 'difficult to present a correct and comprehensive exposition of the extraordinary disease' of hysteria, partly because he had witnessed its manifestation in men, too, even if not 'unequivocally developed'. Usually, though, he found it to be a common symptom of 'deranged menstruation' in women of forty-five and over, and mainly in women 'among the higher and luxurious ranks of society [rather] than among the peasantry – although no class is exempt'.[28] 'With women,' according to the American psychiatrist Isaac Ray (1807–81), 'it is but a short step from extreme nervous susceptibility to downright hysteria, and from that to overt insanity', and in 'sexual evolution . . . strange thoughts, extraordinary feelings . . . criminal impulses, may haunt a mind at other times innocent and pure'.[29] If a woman's virtue and maternal instinct were compromised and her emotional liability proven, she was an obvious case for surgical treatment.

Sexual atrocities were perpetrated on female patients in the name of medicine. Menopausal women who displayed what was considered to be undue sexual excitement or interest were at best ridiculed and at worst subjected to surgery or a spell in the asylum. In his *Psychopathia Sexualis: A medico-forensic study* (1892) the German neurologist Richard von Krafft-Ebing explained that 'in the sedate matron' the loss of sexual desire

is of minor psychological importance, though it is notice-
able. The biological change affects her but little if her sexual
career has been successful, and loving children gladden the
maternal heart. The situation is different, however, where
sterility has denied that happiness, or where enforced
celibacy prevented the performance of natural functions.

Excessive or undue female desire is an ambiguous and, of
course, subjective concept. It wasn't so easily categorized as
drug addiction, kleptomania or homosexuality, being very
much more difficult to define even than these conditions.
Female sexuality itself seemed almost beyond definition. The
existence or otherwise of sexual feeling in women was constantly pontificated upon by medical men. Surgeons such as
William Acton (1813–75) and Isaac Baker Brown (1811–73)
held quite contradictory ideas: Acton believed that most
women had no sexual feeling at all, whilst his colleague
thought otherwise.

Acton was a practising surgeon even though he did not
have a medical degree and was not well thought of by his
peers. A self-nominated expert, he published widely on prostitution, reproductive organs, urology, and male and female
sexuality. 'Happily for society,' he wrote with relief, women
(though not prostitutes) 'know little of or are careless about
sexual indulgences. Love of home, of children, and of domestic duties are the only passions they feel.' Men, on the other
hand, had uncontrollable sexual urges and it was unhealthy
for these to be denied. Baker Brown was a general practitioner and later a surgeon; he knew Sigmund Freud and was
influenced by his ideas on female sexuality, arguing that
women were controlled by their reproductive organs and
that their sexual arousal could lead to disease and insanity.

Marañón took it as read that some menopausal women came to feel a revulsion against the entire male sex, though a few experienced an increase of desire due to 'organic and psychic factors': 'at this age [their] sexual emotions frequently revive and they launch out into love adventures, perhaps for the first time in their lives'.[30] According to the psychiatrist Richard von Krafft-Ebing, women, 'if physically and mentally normal, and properly educated, [have] but little sensual desire . . . the woman who seeks men' is a sheer anomaly.[31] Many in the medical profession damned women with robust sexual appetites as suffering from nymphomania and proposed that they could benefit from the removal of their ovaries, their womb and, sometimes, their clitoris.[32] But there was a real confusion in America, Britain and Europe over the definition of nymphomania. Case histories variously suggested that it was wanting too much coitus or having too much of it, excessive desire, or an overindulgence in masturbation – but who could define excess or lack, or even, really, moderation? C. H. F. Routh, for example, reported that, although older women were not supposed to have any sexual feelings because their ovaries had atrophied, he had performed a cliterodectomy on a woman of seventy-eight who had 'experienced extreme erotic feelings on going to stool', a diagnosis and treatment that brings together a sexually aroused old woman, shame and shit in one heavily taboo-laden idea.[33]

The aetiologies, symptoms and treatments that were bandied about often overlapped with other 'diseases' such as erotomania, hysteria, hystero-epilepsy and ovariomania. Blindness, feelings of strangulation and paralysis were all symptoms associated with hysteria but might also present themselves alongside 'excessive' sexual desire and the patient could be diagnosed as a nymphomaniac suffering with hysteric attacks or a hysteric with nymphomaniacal tendencies, everything depending on the physician's own tendencies. A debate ensued over whether the 'disease' emanated from the brain or the genitals, and while neurologists, anatomists, phrenologists and others looked for an organic cause in the brain, gynaecologists fixed their gaze on the genitals, believing that any 'derangement', such as menopause, could adversely affect the nervous system and the brain and thus result in mental illness.[34]

Isaac Baker Brown, the now infamous member of the Obstetrical Society of London, insisted that insanity resulted from excessive desire and masturbation and recommended clitoridectomy. Surgical excision of the clitoris ('a minor appendage of the genitalia', according to a medical historian in the 1980s)[35] would stop hysteria developing into spinal irritation, and on to idiocy, mania, and even death. He carried out his procedures in a private London clinic for seven years between 1859 and 1866, on children as young as ten, 'idiots', epileptics, paralytics and women with eye problems; five of the operations were performed on women who wanted to take advantage of the 1857 Divorce Act. With spectacularly selective deductive powers he called his surgery a certain cure for nymphomania – he had not been presented with a recurrence of the 'disease' of desire following the procedure. In his work *On the Curability of Certain Forms of Insanity, Epilepsy, Catalepsy, and Hysteria in Females* (London, 1866), Baker Brown includes the case history of a 57-year-old woman: *Case XLVI. Hysterical Homicidal Mania – One Year's Duration – Operation – Cure.*

In December, 1861, Mrs. – came under my care, by the recommendation of Dr Forbes Winslow. She gave me the following history herself:-

History. – she was 57, and had had four children and two
premature labours. The last child was born twenty-three
years ago. Twenty months since had an attack of erysipelas in
the face, with eruptions on different parts of the body. Has
never been well since, and last August had another attack of
erysipelas. Is constantly suffering with shiverings, followed
by burning heat and sweating, with prickling heat of the
skin. For the last year has never slept for more than an hour;
always waking with a *start*; feeling frantic, and very hot and
flushed. Has a constant feeling that she will be lost eternally,
and of this she is constantly speaking.

The woman's husband told Baker Brown that she had begun
to 'show symptoms of mental derangement' a year earlier
and had attempted suicide by trying to jump from a window.
He had his wife confined in an asylum for four months but
she worsened and would wake in the night in a 'frenzy',
'rising up, fighting out with her arms [and in the paroxysm
the desire was always to destroy her husband]'. On examination Baker Brown found her healthy though she would not
look him 'straight in the face', and she 'owned with great
shame to long-continued pernicious habits' of masturbation.
On 14 December, with the husband's connivance, he performed his 'usual operation'. A week later she was sleeping
well but 'will not own to being better' and complained of
'her skin being dry, and "burning hot"'. Baker Brown begged
to differ, saying, on the contrary, that her skin is 'moist and
cool' and, almost wilfully ignoring the hot flushes, recorded
that 'at times she perspires freely'. On 26 December both her
husband and nurse considered her much better but she herself persisted in being, in her doctor's opinion, 'sulky', saying
'she is very bad, and shall soon die'. This poor woman

complained bitterly, too, to Baker Brown's son that his father had 'unsexed her', but he blithely 'answered that nothing of the sort had been done, but that the operation had prevented her from making herself ill'. The woman's husband, on the other hand, was apparently as pleased as punch, calling on the surgeon to thank him for the 'comfort and happiness' he now enjoyed.[36]

It has been powerfully argued that cliterodectomy was the surgical enforcement of an ideology which restricted female sexuality to reproduction. Instinctive and autonomous sexual pleasure, especially after the menopause, was seen as a precipitating cause or a symptom of insanity.[37] Baker Brown was expelled from the Obstetric Society in 1867 after many complaints from patients who felt they had been tricked or coerced into surgery. His colleagues found it difficult to agree on the efficacy or the morality of the procedure, although some regretted its demise. Lawson Tait was almost wistful about its passing, saying, 'I am certain in many cases it could be useful,' and in America there were those who regretted only that Baker Brown's enthusiasm had 'prostituted an occasionally valuable and desirable operation'.[38] Some were a little ambivalent, perhaps, about this incredibly aggressive therapeutic amputation. Some were horrified by it. Wyn Williams thought that the clitoris was probably not the problem, suggesting that the arms and hands were the offending parts and perhaps they should be cut off. Before we congratulate him on his wit, it seems that he did in seriousness think a 'suffering' woman's limbs might be tied behind her back. Seymour Haden, Secretary of the Obstetric Society at the time, condemned it all as a misuse of male power whilst firmly buttressing that hegemony:

we have constituted ourselves, as it were, the guardians of
their interests, and in many cases . . . the custodians of their
honour (*hear, hear*). We are, in fact, the stronger, and they the
weaker. They are obliged to believe all we tell them. They are
not in a position to dispute anything we say to them, and we,
therefore, may be said to have them at our mercy . . . Under
these circumstances, if we should depart from the strictest
principles of honour, if we should cheat or victimize them in
any shape or way, we would be unworthy of the profession of
which we are members (*Loud cheers.*).[39]

William Alcott, American physician and popular medical
writer, bade his colleagues imagine the husband 'who finds
himself united, for life, to a woman whose only defect or
weakness is a slight nymphomania': he might 'think himself
quite fortunate'. And Wells, fully seeing, if not able to bring
himself to completely damn the double standard here, gave
himself up to fancying the

reflected picture of a coterie of Marthas of the profession in
conclave, promulgating the doctrine that most of the
unmanageable maladies of men were to be traced to some
morbid change in their genitals, founding societies for the
discussion of them and hospitals for the cure of them, one of
them sitting in her consultation chair, with her little stove by
her side and her irons all hot, searing every man as he passed
before her.[40]

Another asked, 'would anyone strip off the penis for a stric-
ture or a gonorrhoea, or castrate a man because he had a
hydrocele [an accumulation of fluid in the scrotum] or was a
moral delinquent?' Male patients suffering from satyriasis, a

morbid and overpowering sexual desire in men which corresponded to nymphomania and occurred far less frequently, rarely underwent castration as a cure for their perceived problem. They were the victims of a mild condition, which meant they might be able to learn to control themselves, whilst nymphomaniacs were severely diseased and could end up as depraved prostitutes or in the asylums. Male sexual desire was a norm; men were not defined by their reproductive lives or by their genitalia, and their desires were perceived as emanating from quite different instincts, so castration was never used as a routine treatment for insanity in men.[41] Male sexuality did not threaten the fabric of society in anything like the same way and, if it did, it was the fault of the women they mixed with for either deliberately debauching men or failing to act as a civilizing force and saving them from themselves.

The rare dissenting voice of women, such as that of Elizabeth Garrett Anderson, a political campaigner and the first Englishwoman to qualify as a doctor, asserted that the medical profession distorted female sexuality and diseases. Female sickness was unnecessarily exaggerated and woman's natural functions were just what they were designed to be, and were not abnormal or debilitating. Mary Livermore, a suffrage campaigner, thought it a 'monstrous assumption that woman is a natural invalid' and railed against the 'unclean army of "gynaecologists" who seem desirous to convince women that they possess but one set of organs – and that these are always diseased'. Mary Putnam Jacobi MD wrote in 1895 that 'it is in the increased attention paid to women, and especially in their new function as lucrative patients, scarcely imagined a hundred years ago, that we find explanation for much of the ill-health among women, freshly discovered today'.[42] And Elizabeth Blackwell, daughter of a prominent family of Nonconformists and industrialists in Bristol, England, who graduated as the first female doctor in the US in 1849, thought the 'great increase in ovariotomy, and its extension to the insane is a notable result of this *prurigo secandi* [itch to cut]'.[43] A Dr Currier thought that as 'less than 1% of menopausal women who died in America between 1870 and 1880 had died from cancer of the genital organs', physicians had over-egged the pudding and remained over-influenced by the Ancients.

Ranged against these voices of reason were further counterattacks by male doctors, such as the leading American gynaecologist, Augustus Gardner. In 1872, with a bluntness born of established belief and tradition, he pronounced that women were completely unfit to practise medicine:

> More especially is medicine disgusting for women, accustomed to softness and the downy side of life. They are sedulously screened from the observation of the horrors and disgusts of life. Fightings, and tumults, the blood and mire, bad smells and bad words, and foul men and more intolerable women she but rarely encounters, and then, as a part of the privileges of womanhood, is permitted, and till now, compelled, to avoid them by a not, to her, disgraceful flight.

It is as though Gardner, despite his medical knowledge, could not quite believe that women really bled or defecated or raged. Or if, by some ghastly perversion of sacred nature, they did, 'Male doctors would have to take over the female body for women's own protection.'[44] Robert Barnes was firmly against women entering the medical profession, being better fitted by natural aptitude to the Church where their natural incompatibility with science would do no harm at all.

And the American physician Edward Clarke, Professor of Materia Medica at Harvard College, quoted Henry Maudsley, believing that when a woman has 'pretty well divested herself of her sex – then she may take [male] ground, and do his work, but she will have lost her feminine attractions, and probably also her chief feminine functions' and will be 'thoroughly masculine in nature, or hermaphrodite in mind'.[45]

This united position of firmly established misogyny did not, of course, prevent male doctors from arguing fiercely over the female body amongst themselves. In 1849 a small spat took place in the *Medical Times* between two physicians about who was the first to describe a particular form of 'Climacteric Disease in Women'. Dr Corfe of the Middlesex Hospital had published, on 7 April, a short account of a 'peculiar and important' affection, believing that he was unveiling it for the first time. But on 21 April William Tyler Smith responded, saying he had made a prior claim to the same 'disease' in the Appendix to his work on obstetrics. He was describing hot flushes, 'belonging to the period of "the change of life", or the catamenial crisis', but rather bombastically referred to them as a 'PECULIAR MALADY INCIDENT TO THE DECLINE OF THE CATAMENIA':

The so-called 'heats and chills' of this period consist of a real paroxysmal affection, allied in its nature both to intermittent fever and epilepsy, particularly to the cerebral variety of the latter; sometimes it terminates in epilepsy, or mania, or even apoplexy. In fact, this malady is a fruitful source of mania, occurring in the female after the decline of the catamenia. The disorder I refer to, appears to consist of compression of the vein in the neck, and distention of the cerebral circulation, attended by vivid sensations of heat, flushing of the face and neck, with giddiness, almost amounting to insensibility. These symptoms are soon followed by relaxation of the neck, great coldness or chills, and faintness, with perspiration over the whole of the body. The paroxysms are sometimes so violent as to wake patients out of their sleep, and the apprehensions of the attack produce the greatest uneasiness in excitable patients. The paroxysms occur many times in the twenty-four hours, in women of delicate health, at this epoch. Let any practitioner inquire and analyse the symptoms of women at the catamenial decline, and he will find the affection, of which I have given the outline, to be very common; it is a most important subject of study, as being the basis of many of the disorders of the nervous system which occur after the cessation of the catamenia.[46]

Tyler Smith's recommended treatment for these 'disorders of the nervous system' was sexually barbarous and punitive. To a woman's most delicate tissues he advocated a course of injections of ice water into the rectum, the introduction of ice into the vagina, and the application of leeches to the labia and cervix. His colleagues were advised to count the leeches when they removed them to make sure none was lost and left there. He was coolly impressed by the way the 'suddenness with which leeches applied to this part fill themselves considerably increases the good effects of their application, and for some hours after their removal there is an oozing of blood from the leech-bites'. It must surely have left his patients speechless, though with what emotion it is hard to guess.

The extraordinary barbarity of such men is frankly terrifying, and Lawson Tait, in his *Diseases of Women* (1877), did not disappoint on this score. Tait was a very influential physician whose roles included: Surgeon to Birmingham Hospital for Women; Consulting Surgeon for Diseases of Women to the West Bromwich Hospital; Fellow of the Obstetrical Societies of London, Dublin and Edinburgh; and Foreign Member of the Obstetrical Society of Berlin. He considered menopausal women subject to a set of risks associated with their sexual function which were 'often severe enough to constitute a disease, even though they may have only a subjective existence'. This magnificently vague supposition paved the way for Tait's ideas on some of the general symptoms of the menopause, chief among which were headache and nervous depression. Very few women, he wrote, passed the climacteric period without more or less suffering, and in some cases permanent damage was encountered. The nervous symptoms might be so severe as to result in 'mental derangement', often taking the form of 'incurable dementia'. He had noted in the course of his practice several cases of 'a specific form of climacteric epileptic mania' which he assured his readers was 'entirely irredeemable'. But, worse, he thought the most common and 'I really think the most terrible form of mental disease which is developed at the climacteric, is a tendency to the abuse of alcohol.' Here Tait reveals what is obviously something of a moral mission for him, for a female drinker was secretive and shameful and 'she knows how much more she has to lose than a man has, and how much more misery she will bring upon others'. In woman's defence, and 'in opposition to much clap-trap which it has been of late the fashion to write about their drinking', his 'considerable experience of women who have given themselves up to the habit of intemperance' allows him to say that he has 'never yet had one as a patient in whom there was not some strong inducement to the indulgence'. Many of the women he treated were 'driven to the use of alcoholic anaesthetic by the neglect or infidelity of their husbands; but by far the larger number of these unfortunates have adopted the habit late in life as a relief from their climacteric discomfort'. Seeking oblivion in a bottle from 'some physical suffering [or] mental distress' is 'a form of climacteric insanity', wrote Tait, refusing to believe that 'women ever take to drink from the mere love of it, or from convivial indulgence as men do'. Instead, large numbers of them fell prey to intemperance because they were menopausal, not because their lives were hard or they had large families. It 'would be a wise law', opined the eminent doctor, 'which would enable us to place them in seclusion till the time of their trial is over'. He'd like these menopausal women, who had a drink to escape the difficulties of their lives, locked up.[47]

Tait was a surgeon, a 'blood and guts' man, and he had precious little insight into what he called the 'inner secrets of the mind of a climacteric patient, suffering from such depression as is likely to produce intemperance'. He admitted that he could not broach this subject 'without treading on the province of the alienist [psychiatrist]', but had a go anyway because of the many examples that he considered revealed the 'delusions' of depressed women. He had, for example, case notes of those, believe it or not, who thought they were 'pregnant by men not their husbands'. But 'one of the most terrible was a case in which the poor woman believed that she was pregnant by a dog'. She was removed from home 'without putting her under restraint', her mental occupation was carefully regulated, and within a year her delusions had left her and 'she gave up her intemperate habits completely. The most essential treatment in all these cases is removal from all the former associations of the patient.' This sounds much more like rehab treatment for alcoholism than anything directly attributable to the menopause.

Guy Hinsdale's *Hydrotherapy* (Philadelphia, 1910) suggested that suffering menopausal women were especially good candidates for hydriatic treatment: 'The asthenic physical condition, the mental depression, the irritability, the nervousness, and especially the sleeplessness, are certainly relieved to a great extent by a judicious use of these carbonated saline baths.' Women were enthusiastic about the douche. The use of water as a female masturbatory method is well documented by Shere Hite among others, whereas a jet of pumped water aimed at the male genitalia is more likely to produce pain than pleasure.[48] Tait suggested that menopausal women could be successfully frightened into submission, a technique or 'treatment' that might explain some of the dread and anxiety of women patients and why physicians saw only those who were really suffering. The menopause can make some women stout, he said, and 'they think it is alarming,' or, 'now that tumours are spoken of so much by the public, this dreadful vision . . . is suggested at once, and they appeal for surgical assistance'. He recommended a consultation of two or three practitioners, an examination under anaesthetic and 'the moral force of this proceeding is generally sufficient' to, quite frankly, scare the pants off them.

Many asylums performed routine gynaecological examinations on new female patients. Case reports and admission notes detailed menstrual cycles, their regularity, blood loss and duration. The 'reign of the ovaries [being] undisputed', it was argued that women had a right to the internal examinations as this would, in most cases, reveal the root of their problem. Robert Barnes thought that

not only should women be examined before being commit
ted to asylums ... the asylum authorities should employ
skilled gynaecologists to attend to pelvic disease occurring
among the inmates, *whether or not* the mental condition was
likely to be benefited thereby.[49]

In Tait's opinion the 'relief of nearly all the subjective symptoms of the climacteric period' could best be achieved by the
use of an occasional drastic purgative and, more especially,
'removal from home at frequent intervals'. Shutting troublesome women away certainly had its advocates but the few
women doctors working in asylums generally thought otherwise. Alice May Farnham, an assistant physician at the
Willard Asylum for the Insane in New York, attacked the
popular notion that 'nearly all of those ills to which feminine
flesh is heir' were 'due either to disorders of the female reproductive organs, or so influenced by these organs as to
constitute a peculiar class of diseases'. 'Uterine disease,' she
argued, 'is seldom or never the cause of mental alienation'
and gynaecologists should have no hand in the treatment of
'hysterical, melancholic and maniacal patients'. These
women should remain in the 'grasp' of alienists and neurologists. A New York City neurologist, Louise Robynovitch,
went further, insisting that 'insane women are the legitimate
wards of the woman physician', who was better equipped to
understand her patients' problems as environmental rather
than biological. But female physicians were a minority
whereas female patients were everywhere, and it was thought
that patients with gynaecological problems might find it difficult or shameful to tell male physicians of their conditions
and could even misinterpret any gynaecological treatment
they received, thereby exacerbating their mental illness.

Amelia Gilmore, resident physician at the Insane Department of the Philadelphia Hospital, suggested that 'the tendency to eroticism is not provoked when the patients are under the medical care of women' and, radically, by the end of the century, several states had passed laws to provide female care for female patients.[50]

The editor of *Alienist and Neurologist* complained in 1882 that the typical woman patient has 'the imaginary notion that her womb is diseased', one reporting that she 'had a feeling, which many women I know also have, that the womb is the weak point and is the cause of most of their nervous ills'. Dr Lilian Welsh knew there was scarcely a woman patient of hers 'with a neurotic history or a neurotic tendency whose mind was not fixed upon her reproductive organs as the source of all her troubles', and a colleague was 'continually asked by the friends of the insane, "Is there not some uterine trouble?"'; 'people,' she continued, 'think that all mental disorder springs from uterine trouble. They forget that there are more insane men than women, so the uterus cannot be held responsible for all insanity.' But the apparent ease with which it could be whipped out must have fed the hope that madness could be quickly and effectively fixed, and the most popular form of surgery performed on nervous and insane women was the removal of one or both ovaries.[51]

The ancient idea of the uterus exerting autonomous, controlling force over the body was giving way to the nervous system as a new explanatory medical diagnosis. Victorian psychiatry, like Victorian gynaecology, saw its work with females as a fight to stabilize their minds against almost overwhelming odds. Woman was both a 'product and prisoner of her reproductive system', and all there was to know of her, all her virtues and depravities, her glories and deformities, continued to radiate from that source. Her status as 'a moral, a sexual, a germiferous, gestative, and parturient creature' was ably and repeatedly demonstrated by the findings of science, according to Charles Meigs in 1847, when he lectured his medical students at Jefferson Medical College on some of the distinctive characteristics of the female. The 'functions of the brain are so intimately connected with the uterine system, that the interruption of any one process which the latter has to perform in the human economy may implicate the former'.[52]

The matron of the first American purpose-built women's prison (a section of Mount Pleasant Prison in New York, popularly known as Sing Sing), Eliza Farnham, campaigned for the recognition and use of the new psychology of phrenology, the study of the skull to deduce mental faculties and character, to diagnose and cure female prisoners. A social reformer and advocate of suffrage, she knew 'that many a woman has experienced, at times, a secret joy in her advancing age', that post-menopausal years could be ones of 'super-exaltation', and she condemned the idea that the menopause was an 'absolutely uncompensated loss of power'. Comparing a woman's life with a man's, Farnham argued that the latter was physiologically divided into two stages, youth and maturity, whilst the former was much more complex and had three stages: ante-maternal, maternal and post-maternal. In the post-maternal stage the world could see the evidence of 'the superiority of woman'.[53]

Most women who found themselves as inmates in prisons and asylums, however, were said to be suffering from a derangement of their reproductive life. They 'may become insane if the menstrual flux hang about in the head in lieu of taking its proper course' and some felt that a 'Genuine

Insanity is CANCER OF THE MIND'.[54] This disease, though, was often accompanied by 'disappointment' or 'family troubles', whilst male insanity was most often assigned causes such as overwork, business worries, self-abuse and debauchery, all of which miseries reflect traditional sex roles and expectations.[55] Climacteric insanity was often stated explicitly as the exciting cause of the madness: Elinor D., aged forty-six, was admitted to Pen-y-Fal asylum following a 'reversal of fortune' in her family situation and her own subsequent suicide attempt and the cause given was 'probably climacteric'; Frances D., aged forty-eight, was admitted in a distressed and bruised state and her problems were also recorded as 'Cause said to be climacteric'. There was no record of an investigation into her physical injuries.

Displays of sullenness, nervousness, depression, insecurity, wildness, excitement and volubility were easily attributed to a menopausal woman's position in society. Queen Victoria herself was not immune to suspicions that she might be insane, especially because of the extent and nature of her grief on losing her husband. Her physician, Sir William Jenner, gave medical authority to the opinion that she was incapable of making public appearances, and her household found 'extreme difficulty . . . in managing her or in the slightest degree contradicting her'. During the 1860s, when she was in her fifth decade, rumour and gossip over her state of mind were the subject of many politicians' conversations and letters. They were facing the perceived dangers of a woman on the throne without the appropriate, rational and necessary control of a husband. Her naturally self-willed, opinionated and proud character placed her under suspicion. The fears faded away once she had gone through her menopause.[56]

Gender and age influenced the diagnosis, confinement and treatment of any woman seen as labouring under what was increasingly a panoply of mental disorders. Older women were considered to have been stripped of their 'glorifying maternal function', the ultimate aim of their existence nullified and, with it, the sexual self. For, if sex was procreation then desire must die, because if not it would mean that women had their own sexuality and might be dangerously independent of reproduction. Either that or they could become 'shadows of the shadows which they already were', sinking into a melancholy and powerless mental state often diagnosed as 'lypemania'. The relationship between madness and menopause was considered very close but was understood as a derangement of the reproductive system rather than a consequence of a loss of status and value, both emotional and economic.[57]

W. A. F. Brown, in his study *What Asylums Were, Are, and Ought to Be* (New York, 1837), went so far as to argue that 'in the case of a public asylum, a larger portion of the building should be allotted to females, as their numbers almost always predominate'. George Man Burrows, in *Commentaries on Insanity* (1828), reasoned similarly on the grounds that 'The functions of the brain are so intimately connected with the uterine system, that the interruption of any one process which the latter has to perform in the human economy may implicate the former.' According to G. Fielding Blandford, who in 1894 was president of the psychiatric section of the British Medical Association, 'Women become insane during pregnancy, after parturition, during lactation; at the age when the catamenia first appear and when they disappear.' The 'sympathetic connection' existing between the brain and the reproductive organs, 'plainly seen by the most casual observer', was a 'special law', whatever that might be. According to Horatio R. Storer, in his book *The Causation, Cause, and Treatment of Reflex Insanity in Women* (1871), it consisted of women being 'the victims of periodicity' and led to a distinct set of mental illnesses that had 'neither homologue nor analogue in man'.[58] Manias, neuroses and 'ovarian insanity' extending into senescence were the lot of those whose 'periodicity' ceased, as 'Nature,' opined C. C. Hersman in 1899, 'just before the change of life, takes revenge for too severe repression of all manifestations of sex – this may take a turn similar to nymphomania . . . the beginning and end of a very sad picture.'

Even women who were not actually insane were quite likely to offer 'insane interpretations' of their menopausal symptoms, according to George Savage, writing in the *Lancet* in 1903, whilst others suggested that popular notions of hysteria educated women into that behaviour and held women complicit in the creation of the ovaries as a 'bogy which cast its shadow over any or all parts of the body'. It would be 'as easy to remove Helvellyn and plant it in Wicklow as to remove the impression produced on her mind'.[59]

Rees Philips, a medical superintendent at Holloway Sanatorium, 'acknowledged that women are more prone to insanity than men'. In June 1886, Alice, a married woman aged forty-five, was admitted to his institution with 'hysterical mania', said to be caused by the onset of her menopause, there being no obvious physical problem or change apart from this. Alice's 'crisis', exacerbated by a trip to Spain, had caused her to jump out of a window, the first of several suicide attempts she subsequently made after her incarceration. So distressed was she that she took to banging her head repeatedly against the walls, screamed continuously, tried to gouge out her eyes and bit her lips until she looked 'a ghastly subject with her lips swollen beyond recognition and eyes the colour of claret'. They injected her with morphia, administered purgatives, gave her electric therapy and regularly dispatched her to their seaside residence for short visits.[60] Having shown herself to be a 'ghastly subject', Alice had compounded her faults, for interest in one's appearance was viewed as sane whilst neglect was a sign of insanity, this despite the fact that 'excessive' vanity, whatever that was deemed to be, was also a form of madness. Where the line was drawn between care and neglect was, of course, subjective and cultural.

If hysteria had a psychological basis then, *pace* Freud, if women could lose their neurosis their menopausal symptoms would disappear.[61] But, less than a decade after Jean-Martin Charcot's death in 1893 and the publication of *Studies on Hysteria* by Freud and Breuer, came the first statement by a medical author on the decline of the disease. In 1907 Armin Steyerthal, director of a private health spa in Germany, asked, 'What is hysteria?' and predicted that 'within a few years the concept of hysteria will belong to history . . . there is no such disease and there never has been'. The *belle époque* of the disease in the closing years of the nineteenth century turned into its virtual disappearance two decades later, but not before hordes of women were diagnosed and treated for it.

In 1914, Paul Giraud, an asylum doctor in Tours, France, writing in the *Annales Médico-Psychologiques*, mooted that 'for some time now one has no longer dared to speak of hysteria. Multiple theories clash and typical cases have become rarer and rarer.'[62] The poets Louis Aragon and André Breton, in one of their surrealist manifestos in 1928, hailed hysteria as 'the greatest poetic discovery of the late nineteenth century', yet a year later Marañón published his weighty work in England taking the diagnosis of hysteria very seriously indeed as far as the menopausal woman was concerned. Positing a new link between the womb and the brain, he described an exciting phase of instability 'through which most women pass in the first stages of the climacteric', and proposed that this acted 'unfavourably on hysteria'. On the other hand, when the menopause was complete and there was 'definite suppression of the ovary . . . the symptoms lessen and even disappear'. He cited the case of N. R., a female patient, 'always hysteric with severe typical manifestations throughout life, exacerbated by an abnormal sexual life': in her forty-second year she suffered 'an aggravation of all her symptoms . . . sensations of heat and other menopausal manifestations. Then the *hysteric phenomena were intensified extraordinarily*; attacks, oppressions and varying paralyses, [her] digestion was impaired; hysteric psychology greatly exaggerated.' This turbulent period lasted two years, then, 'parallel to the subsidence of the menopausal crisis, a *progressive lessening of the hysteria began*. Now five months have passed without menses and the hysteria clinically has completely disappeared [original emphasis].' Marañón noted that 'cases have also been cited wherein hysterism appeared for the first time in the physiologic menopause, in women who had been healthy until then, or after an early menopause, or even following castration' – though not as a cause but probably as a latent hysteria being revealed by menopause.[63]

The hysterical tide continued to turn, however, and by 1949 Georges Guillain was explaining, in *La semaine des hôpitaux*, that 'in reality, the patients have not changed since Charcot; it is the words to describe them that have changed'. After

2500 years of acceptance of the disease, no physician was quite sure what it was. In 1953 George Swetlow, a professor of medico-legal jurisprudence in New York, suggested that it was a 'strange disorder in that it takes a position mid-way between truth and deceit – not only may hysterical symptoms caricature almost any known disability due to actual tissue alteration, but at the same time it presents features hardly distinguishable from fraud', explaining everything and therefore nothing. Psychiatric diseases go in and out of fashion more than do the diseases of other branches of medical science, depending on the Zeitgeist, and hysteria collapsed under the weight of the many clinical states that it appeared to contain. Many cases of hysteria are now believed to have involved physical diseases such as epilepsy, syphilis, multiple sclerosis and cranial injury.[64]

A ponderously persistent belief in the almost mystical power of the ovary had rubbed shoulders with a scientific connection between the organ and everyday female functions. The ovary's apparent influence over the soul of women was now seen to have a direct effect on their minds and behaviour. The heavy-handed use of surgical procedures and treatments tried to damp down what passed for unnatural, unfeminine behaviour. Sex, the key to women's difference and difficulty, could be extirpated. But not all physicians were so dogmatically definite: Henry Park Newman, Professor of Gynaecology at Chicago Medical School in the 1890s, stressed that 'woman must be more than the material upon which to exploit skill in perfecting radical and often mutilating operations'. One should know 'as much about women as about disease; as much about environmental and social and domestic conditions as about pelvic lesions; as much about causes as about results'.[65] His was a voice of reason pitted against an embedded understanding of women's difference, but it also emphasized that unruly otherness in women and the need for their containment and modification. Attempting to explain and solve the perceived difficulty of women by regulating them and trying to bring them into line with the orderly male body was a doomed enterprise. The friction between ideas of passivity, modesty and domesticity, and the demands for education and increasing numbers of working women only aggravated the opposition of the sexes.

6

SEX, SCIENCE AND SENSIBILITY

'Don't offer them flowers, gentlemen. Offer them estrogen!'[1]

With a nifty bit of faint if lurid praise, Jules Michelet had damned the female sex as doing 'nothing as we do'. In *Women's Love and Life* (1881) he categorized them as such a long way short of the ideal as to be almost another species. Writing for his own sex he described womankind as, at the very least, a distinctly other creature to man, one who

> thinks, speaks, and acts differently. Her tastes are different from our tastes. Her blood even does not flow in her veins as ours does, at times it rushes through them like a foaming mountain torrent. She does not respire as we do. Making provision for pregnancy and the future ascension of the lower organs, nature has so constructed her that she breathes, for the most part, by the four upper ribs. From this necessity, results woman's greatest beauty, and gently undulating bosom, which expresses all her sentiments by a mute eloquence. She doesn't eat like us — neither as much nor of

the same dishes. Why? Chiefly, because she doesn't digest as
we do. Her digestion is every moment troubled by one thing.
She yearns with her very bowels. The deep cup of love
(which is called the pelvis) is a sea of varying emotions, hin-
dering the regularity of the nutritive functions.[2]

Michelet believed that a woman's existence was dictated by
her body, she didn't need to speak even, as her breasts could
do that for her, saying all that was apparently necessary to
say. Unlike man, she had little to express or offer apart from
her reproductive function, a supposition that puts post-
menopausal women firmly in their place at the bottom of
the heap. Her 'difference' was undoubtedly seen as a major
problem, a puzzle requiring a solution. When defined by
comparison with a male 'ideal', there was something essentially wrong with her. Hence the idea that she could be
somehow 'fixed'.

Menopause took women further still from even an ideal
femininity – if they couldn't be like men they could at least
be a perfect fit for men. A woman who flouted what was prescribed as 'true' femininity, one who committed adultery,
flirted or felt more passionate than her husband, even
women who got divorced, could be diagnosed as diseased.
Menopause, in robbing a woman of femininity, invited disease
and might drive her to violence, suicide, drugs, drink and
sex (and if that doesn't sound like someone breaking out or
rebelling, it's hard to say what does). But, if she behaved herself and got through her menopause safely with the 'sweet
consciousness of duty performed', she could smugly 'sur-
round herself with a saintly halo of kind words' and then,
knowing her place, quietly and without any more undue fuss
'pass onwards to the silence of eternal rest'.[3]

Some commentators were beginning to realize that femaleness could not be fixed and static, could not be so easily categorized, but was a constantly changing social concept outside of the question of biology.[4] 'We have not succeeded in determining the radical and essential characters of men and women uninfluenced by external modifying conditions,' reasoned Havelock Ellis in *Man and Woman* (1894). A writer on the psychology of sex, he understood that

> We have to recognise that our present knowledge of men and women cannot tell us what they might be or what they ought to be, but what they actually are, under the conditions of civilisation. By showing us that under varying conditions men and women are, within certain limits, indefinitely modifiable, a precise knowledge of the actual facts of the life of men and women forbids us to dogmatise rigidly concerning the respective spheres of men and women.

This discussion of sex difference, even 'sex antagonism', was happening at a time of rapid advances and great optimism in medical research. In the late nineteenth century, alongside the introduction of anaesthesia, antisepsis and germ-theory, there was research into the secretions of endocrine glands such as the thyroid, adrenals, ovaries and testicles. Even while this early experimental work on human hormones in the 1890s was being carried out, physicians were still debating the role of ovaries, wondering whether the uterus was an independent organ, or if menstruation was provoked by the Fallopian tubes.[5] Walter Heape, a British physiologist and the first to study the human menstrual cycle in relation to the oestrus cycle in animals, published his book *Sex Antagonism* in 1913. This anthropological study, arguing that women's biological destiny was directly opposite to men's, allowed him to refute roundly the increasingly loud call for equal rights. A woman's destiny, proclaimed Heape, was restricted to motherhood by virtue of her biology and that was that. The Viennese gynaecologist Eugen Steinach had attached the idea of sex antagonism to the concept of sex hormones and also argued for the established cultural differences between the sexes. Popular commentators took up and supported these apparently irrefutable 'facts': 'the chemical war between the male and the female hormones is, as it were, a chemical miniature of the well-known eternal war between men and women'. Sex antagonism was one 'weapon' in the 'war' against a nascent women's liberation movement.[6]

In 1905 Martha Covey Thomas, president of the women's liberal arts college Bryn Mawr in Pennsylvania, responded with fierce pithiness to the view of psychologist G. Stanley Hall of women as slaves to the workings of their reproductive system. Now we know, she said, that it is not woman but man who believes 'such things about us, who is himself pathological, blinded by the neurotic mists of sex, unable to see that women form one-half of the kindly race of normal, healthy creatures in the world'. The scientific facts were not facts at all, according to the American psychologist Leta Stetter Hollingworth, they were merely literary traditions carried on by mystics and romantics. Their sentimental prose had found its way into medical texts which validated ideas of woman as a 'mysterious being, half hysteric, half angel'. Healthy women did not approach alienists, physicians, obste-tricians and gynaecologists, only hysterics, women with mental and physical diseases, came under the medical gaze.[7] Medicine misunderstood womankind as a whole.

Where nineteenth-century women attempted to shake off

cultural restraints they were accused, like menopausal women, of transgressing against nature and not just society· their movements were seen as muscular and less womanly, where they had been quiet and graceful, they were abrupt and direct. Their voices grew louder, their tones more assertive, and they would insist on speaking out, leaving nothing to the imagination. This alleged biological regression was said to reduce women to sexless substitutes for men. To attack women's sex, when sex was all they were supposed to be, was considered the worst insult – but these women knew they were more than their biology and could continue their struggle for emancipation strengthened by the spurious logic of their detractors.

Vile gynophobia was nothing new, of course. Charles Meigs, in *Females and Their Diseases* (1848), had castigated women for 'dereliction of duty', warning them that bad behaviour and subverting nature would surely be punished. Bitterness would be visited upon them like a proper plague of boils. Purity movement writers took up this argument, claiming to measure the extent of discomfort and disease by the degree of abuse a woman had subjected herself to. They blamed the frequency and seriousness of disease during and after menopause upon 'indiscretions' committed in youth – a hell on earth. Older women could only suffer and be contrite, younger ones still had time to curtail their behaviour and save themselves. They were warned about any excess in sexual passion, dress, stimulating foods, prurient reading material, contraception and the 'solitary vice' of masturbation; all of these were said to increase the hardships a woman might suffer later at her leisure. The *Ladies Guide in Health and Disease. Girlhood, Maidenhood, Wifehood, Motherhood* (1883), written by the American surgeon John Kellogg with an evangelical belief in divine connections between health and morality, preached that women who 'transgressed nature's laws' would find the menopause a 'veritable Pandora's box of ills, and may well look forward to it with apprehension and foreboding'. Women writing on the menopause were often complicit in the hell-fire and fear-mongering. Emma Francis Angell Drake for one had baldly stated in her book *What a Woman of Forty-Five Ought to Know* (1902), published when she was fifty-two, that 'many things that have been laid to our ancestors remotely distant are really the result of wrongdoing and living in the first decade and a half of our lives'. Nature, personified as female and as an unforgivingly cruel avenging god, will rebel and compel the 'payment of her violated laws', usually with an onslaught of malignant disease or, 'failing this, a slow and dangerous change is likely to be experienced, followed by years of discomfort or invalidism'.[8]

Treatments to circumvent menopausal miseries that were waiting to hit mid-life women were in the offing, and women themselves were involved in the early experiments with glandular extracts. One Parisian midwife was reported to have given herself liquid made from pigs' ovaries with beneficial effects. The prolific British-born French physiologist and neurologist Charles-Édouard Brown-Séquard thought that the ovaries of animals would yield an extract which had the same effect on women as his testicular extract purportedly had on men. He regarded hot flushes as curiosities and couldn't decide whether they were normal or morbid but knew that some essence, 'an unknown quantity', lay behind them. All things considered, though, he inclined to the view that 'they are not normal' and needed treatment. He reported on an American doctor, Augusta Brown, who had given more than a dozen older women the 'filtered juice of guinea-pigs' ovaries with good effect in cases of hysteria, in various uterine infections, and in debility due to age'. This was confirmed in a report by the physician H. R. Andrews in 1904, who noted forty-six such experiments on women but, he said, 'without much success'. A Marseille surgeon, Dr Villeneuve, used this method on two women; one, he recorded, 'who suffered with hysterical seizures following oophorectomy, was cured'.[9] Compton Burnett also used hormone extracts when his own homeopathic medicines failed. For hot flushes he prescribed Lachesis, Glonoin and Urtica urens, but if the flushes were severe he used ovarian extract. Some women obviously had faith in this work. A Miss C., aged fifty-two, who suffered from haemorrhages and violent, frequent flushes, allowed him to plug her vagina and administer iced injections on removal of the plugs twice daily. She also took ergot, arsenic, potassium bromide, calcium chloride, thyroid gland extract and five-grain doses of ovarian gland three times a day. After a period of treatment Compton Burnett claimed her cured.[10]

This was the early vision of endocrinology, the study of the glands of internal secretion and their role in the physiology of the body. In practice it was the testing of 'ill defined extracts on hysterical women'[11] – the beginning of the use of drugs to try to change the nature of the female sex. In the 1890s, Viennese scientists had established the existence of ovarian hormones and in the early twentieth century Edward Sharpey-Schafer (1850–1935) laid down the physiological foundations of endocrinology. F. H. A. Marshall (1878–1949) and William Jolly (1873–1945) made detailed investigations of ovarian endocrinology within general biology rather than as a special interest to gynaecologists. They explored the female cycle in domestic animals (the ewe, ferret and bitch) but not in women, whose cycles 'were still imperfectly understood by the puzzled clinicians'.[12] The secretions, known as 'hormones', were named on the suggestion of a Cambridge classicist, from the Greek 'I excite', and the term was first used in Britain in 1905 by Ernest H. Starling, Professor of Physiology at University College London. 'These chemical messengers,' he said,

> or 'hormones' as we may call them, have to be carried from the organ where they are produced to the organ which they affect, by means of the blood stream, and the continually recurring physiological needs of the organism must determine their production and circulation through the body.[13]

A decade later Sir William Maddock Bayliss wrote in his *Principles of General Physiology* about 'a large number of substances, acting powerfully in minute amount, which are of great importance in physiological processes'. The hormones,

> or chemical messengers, which are produced in a particular organ, pass into the blood current and produce effects in different organs. They provide, therefore, for a chemical co-ordination of the activities of the organism, working side by side with that through the nervous system.

After 1910 the existence of sex hormones was no longer being seriously questioned and discussion centred only on the best method of their study, definition, isolation, assay and possible synthesis.[14] This was considered an heroic age of reproductive endocrinology. In America the Association for the Study of Internal Secretions was founded in June 1917, becoming the Endocrine Society in 1952, when it was suggested that early hostility towards their work meant that it might have been safer to have met in secret. Edward Doisy, a biochemist, and Edgar Allen, a zoologist, had devised the criteria which established it as an acceptable field of scientific study by 1936. Ovarian hormones were now being isolated and synthesized: oestrin in 1923, progesterone in 1929, oestriol in 1930, oestrone in 1930 and oestradiol in 1936.[15]

Hormone after hormone was coming to light and the workings of the endocrine system revealed, and with this new knowledge came ideas and assumptions about human minds, bodies and, not least, morals.[16] Sex difference, and what made a man a man and a woman a woman, began to seem, for the first time since Aristotle, like an indisputable scientific reality. Men and women were opposites rather than complementary creatures. Yet at the same time, it was now thought potentially possible that men and women could escape their biology by manipulating these hormones, and all this was happening during a period when cultural and political ideas on eugenics, race and heredity were gaining ground and popularity.

Eugen Steinach, an influential Viennese physiologist working at the turn of the twentieth century, believed that, by irradiating their hormones, he could rejuvenate and restore the 'femininity' that he considered older women had lost. The American novelist Gertrude Atherton tried it when she had writer's block and claimed that the eight sessions of X-rays directed at her ovaries caused her torpor to vanish. Her brain, she gushed, 'seemed sparkling with light' and she threw herself into writing *Black Oxen* (1923), a hugely successful novel about female rejuvenation. After the American biochemist Louis Berman published the extraordinarily popular *The Glands Regulating Personality* in 1921, the *New York Times* proclaimed that a 'war-ridden world' had been succeeded by a 'gland-ridden' one, even though the science was new and fraught with uncertainties.[17]

Not everyone was quite so enthusiastic about all this progress. Marañón believed that the 'astonishing experiments of the last few years' which had established the possibility of realizing therapeutic rejuvenation by 'ligating the epididymis or the vas deferens in man or by ovarian roentgenotherapy in woman, or by transplanting the genital glands of apes' were verging on outright quackery. He panned the over-excited claims, dismissing them as 'limited to a passing reactivation of a sexual function which was languishing, and to an equally mild and transitory reanimation of the general state'. They were, in effect, a 'sham', and the paucity and inconstancy of the results meant he could not condone the 'treatments'. In his opinion the ovarian grafts, known as opotherapy, would just be absorbed by the body and lost, and the commercial preparations were a complete con. These extracts were delivered by subcutaneous injection or by mouth, and consisted of either 'whole extract of the ovary' or 'preparations of *corpus luteum*', dessicated or glycerinated. With growing irritation he admonished the purveyors as 'childish' in seeking to give a general dose to women; any such substance should be attuned to the individual and would vary over time. Yet, despite his reservations and even though he knew that the medical knowledge 'remains vague', he could still recommend that it be used on menopausal women, claiming that the 'results of ovarian therapy in the climacteric are excellent, in general', though how he measured or justified this is uncertain.

The menopause, wrote Marañón, was a biologic consequence of an 'endocrine crisis which varies in different individuals'; it was not 'merely a syndrome of genital insufficiency', though this was a fundamental element. The 'classic concept of the *menopause* as a simple genital incident in woman' was nonsense. He believed in the complex transitional syndrome which implicated other organs and systems within the body. It was an excitingly complex 'pluriglandular interpretation'. He thought this was 'doubtless one of the great contributions of endocrinology to biology within the last twenty years' but, in fact, it mirrors past ways of understanding the menopause, such as Fothergill's, and was merely expressing the same ideas in a modern, scientific language.

A menopausal woman's physical and emotional life deviated, Marañón continued, 'on minor stimuli, from the normal', becoming 'exquisitely sensitized'. He dubbed it the 'age of emotion' – when a woman is prone to irrationality and 'an increase of emotional attacks'. Menopause and emotion were 'two inseparable factors' and the individual's temperament would determine her experience. The 'virile', 'bold' and 'energetic' woman will suffer, he says, more than the 'very "womanly" woman – those who are delicate, fragile, childish'. This is a modern version of the old humoural theory, with hormones replacing humours and similar assumptions of character and type underlying them.

Lauding hormonal therapy in France in the 1930s, Dr Pauchet held menopause to be 'a veritable psychological crisis' when a woman altered her 'physiognomy, external appearance, voice, and even character', which meant she might become 'cantankerous' – instead of meek, mild and biddable presumably. She could become far too manly physically, as 'virile cells take on such importance that the face acquires a masculine aspect: the nose lengthens, the hair of the cheeks, upper lip, and chin become a beard'.[18] Boundaries between 'maleness' and 'femaleness' began to seem more malleable, but cultural mores were harder to shift. In 1938 Marius Tausk, the medical director of the pharmaceutical company Organon in the 1920s and 30s, was amazed at the experimental treatment of menopausal women with male sex hormones and, although treatment with testosterone allegedly produced striking results, he didn't believe it would replace 'the known hormonal therapy of menopause with ovarian hormone'. A Dutch gynaecologist working in the 1940s was of the firm opinion that, as women were 'controlled' by the hormonal functioning of their ovaries, they were subject to a 'major physiological and bodily lability', a 'problem' which did not exist for men, and this 'is the reason why women are handicapped in their struggle for equality with men'.[19]

The potent mix of science, of educational, emotional and social influences, had thrown everything into confusion in the 1920s and 30s. Bernhard Zondek (1891–1966) had found small quantities of oestrone in the urine of human males and discovered that the urine of pregnant mares was another rich source, a finding which led to commercialization.[20] Then, even more remarkable to many, came the news that the testes of stallions contain 500 times more oestrone than the ovaries of mares. As Starling remarked, 'Who could have expected that the gonads of a male animal would turn out to be the richest source of female sex hormone ever observed?' In 1965, just before the 'Summer of Love', it was wryly suggested that the present wonder was that the 'balance of endocrine factors usually come down on one side or the other to produce a recognisable male or female – perhaps in these days, I should say, a more or less recognisable male or female'. Presentation is perhaps 90 per cent of the argument.

Science was giving another dimension of meaning to sex difference and cultural notions of masculinity and femininity with an arguably uncritical acceptance of female and male sex hormones as natural fact. But there was some dissent from those who felt that they had not found sex hormones simply 'somewhere in a lost corner, like a desert island lost in the mist'. They had themselves 'called sex hormones into existence' and made of them a material reality. This had bestowed on chemical substances a sexual identity of their own based on traditional ideas of ovaries as the essence of femininity.[21]

The manufacture of the first synthetic 'oestrogen', stilboestrol, was quickly followed by another, dynestrol. These preparations could be manufactured economically by the kilogram, but a connection between their use and cancer was recognized very early in the research. The Radium Institute in Paris induced carcinomas in male mice which had been injected with female sex hormones. The findings were obviously detrimental to promoting and selling the preparations – and they were downplayed. Smaller doses were prescribed, using the old argument that we wouldn't stop using salt just because it is deadly in large quantities. By 1939 reports on the increased incidence of breast cancer following injections with the first synthetic female sex hormone, known as DES, were published, but the drugs continued to be promoted and the positive effects emphasized despite their largely unknown qualities and the nascent research. The idea of the 'hormonal female' was formed as the science was married to traditional cultural and institutional attitudes to women.[22]

Many of the doctors who were publishing papers in American medical journals between 1938 and 1941 had experimented with DES and, as part of the US medical elite, their influence formed the basis of the government's decision about the safety of DES. Science, they thought, would help medicine become safer and at the same time served to increase medicine as a cultural authority. DES was considered an efficacious drug but disagreements about its safety began to be aired as some patients were suffering from nausea, vomiting and skin rashes. But by 1941 most specialists thought it safe based on clinical observations – studies that relied almost exclusively on those women who were seeking medical help for their menopausal symptoms, ignoring all others. When oestrogen deficiency was used as the sole explanation of menopausal symptoms it reduced the experiences of ageing women to biologically determined problems and reinforced the traditional view of women as different and inferior. Hormone replacement therapy (HRT) became not only legitimate but almost obligatory. The underlying message was that all menopausal women would be mad or irresponsible not to seek medical attention to correct themselves.[23]

Women who wanted to try the drugs might face another uphill struggle here, though, attempting to convince those disinterested and unimpressed doctors who still laboured 'under the false idea that woman should endure it'.[24] Elizabeth Parker, in *The Seven Ages of Women* (1960), produced a strong argument for medical intervention. She knew that there was, in fact, much that medicine could, and *should*, do, even though her ideas were neither radical nor new but echoed her medical predecessors in all previous centuries. Menopause was, she said, 'different for every woman. There is no fixed pattern, no chain of events that must transpire. The onset is imperceptible, the end unpredictable, the duration indefinite, and the experience different for every woman' who approached her menopause 'with reluctance and sometimes with fear because of the many misconceptions, myths, and superstitions that are passed on to her'. But 'nothing could be more untrue or more absurd' than to suggest that her emotional life would dry up, or that she risked losing her mind, having a nervous breakdown or sinking into melancholia because her menstrual function ceased. A woman was not 'more susceptible to any disease', though 'she can, of course, have any of the illnesses to which flesh is heir . . . but not because she is in the Age of the Menopause'. Parker's 'new' angle was a broader concept: 'the Age of Serenity'. And to achieve this ghastly implication of enforced tranquillity, like it or not, a woman must go to 'the only person who can give her facts, her doctor, who will reassure and guide her in the solution of her problem'.

Self-help was essential and fundamental, but self-medication was dangerous and best left to the experts: 'there are things only her doctor can and *should* do for her'. For hot flushes, upon which she had to admit, 'doctors are not quite agreed', the important thing was to have your share of 'the estrogenic hormone'. Indeed, Parker never ceased 'to marvel at what a few drops of a certain liquid in a syringe or even a few gaily colored tablets can mean to the well-being and happiness of a woman'. It all rested on the endocrine glands because the 'ovaries go to sleep' – much like your socks did when you were a little girl.

Parker made great claims: advances were 'spectacular', the treatment of menopause had been revolutionized and hormone treatment had changed the 'whole concept of the meaning of the menopause': it could stabilize women's personalities. She made no mention of the synthetic nature of the chemicals used or the different amounts administered. Modern woman was a demanding woman and was 'indeed fortunate' to be able to obtain relief from any unpleasant symptoms. The purpose was to 'smooth the transition, not to delay or defer it, and certainly not to prolong it'. The infallible doctor could be called upon to inject the dotty menopausal woman with the magic oestrogen, it being 'so easy to forget to take the tablet'. An injection was a controlled 'reservoir from which the hormone is liberated slowly over . . . three or four days to two weeks or a month . . . a smooth and prolonged action' and treatment should be individualized. The fag of going regularly to the doctor and the expense involved were worth it as he would be 'alert to untoward side effects or over-dosage'. A woman in charge of her own prescribed tablets is worryingly out of his control and 'out of his hands'. The hormone preparations relieved the 'anxiety and depression of menopause but also restored a feeling of well-being', whereas tranquillizers only masked the need for them. A woman's problems too were lessened, not because she could effectively ignore them, but because she would feel 'fit to meet them with courage and determination'.

Eventually Parker got round to asking, in upper case, 'ARE HORMONES DANGEROUS?' Acknowledging that women have heard that hormones cause cancer, make facial hair grow and do not relieve the menopause but only delay or prolong it, Parker admitted that 'some hormones do have some relationship to the growth (not cause) of cancer'. In the early days 'when estrogen first became available for use in potent amounts, too much was used and unwanted side effects were produced'. Women given androgen had developed a fuzzy growth of hair on the face, an acne that was worse than they had experienced in adolescence, their voices became husky and they 'quickly spread the word that hormones caused symptoms that were worse than hot flashes', though all unwanted signs disappeared when the hormones were stopped, merely indicating that more careful regulation of dosage was the answer. Though 'no one can say with certainty that hormones do or do not cause cancer', Parker argued that oestrogen had been accused of complicity in the crime on circumstantial evidence, which is far from sufficient to convict. Yet 'the stigma has persisted' despite women naturally having oestrogen in their bodies which has benefited them, and which was at times present in very high levels, depending on their life cycle. Still, her message was always necessarily qualified. Oestrogen, she said, was a 'growth hormone' and stimulated growth in tissues sensitive to it, particularly the uterus or breasts, and as cancer cells in those organs 'might be stimulated to grow faster . . . doctors are reluctant to give estrogen to women known to have had cancer in the breast or the uterus'.

The menopausal woman was weighed down with 'cancer-fear, with impending nervousness, or craziness, but most often with the basic dread of loss of femininity and sexual attractiveness, or changes in the body image', according to Dr J. Romano in the 1960s. This 'cancer-fear' is a curious turn-around as by far the greatest terror of the disease at this time was produced by emerging stories around the use of HRT. Now it was being described as a menopausal symptom.[25] Penny Wise Budoff reported in 1976 that many of her patients had benefited from HRT – sleeping better, taking fewer tranquillizers, continuing an active sex life and even undergoing 'profound personality changes' – but she was cautious, suggesting screening and monitoring, and counselling that if they were 'still fearful' of the cancer risk they should not take the drugs. 'If you want estrogen forever,' she wrote, 'because you are sedentary, thin, white, and fear for your bones, that's fine.'[26]

Caution was becoming more prevalent, however. Joseph Rogers, in *Endocrine and Metabolic Aspects of Gynaecology* (1963), worried about the considerable variation between women and wondered whether the menopause was so difficult to understand and treat because it was a biologic accident which had come about because of increased life expectancy, conveniently ignoring the menopause in history. He believed that the only hormonally mediated symptoms of the menopause were disrupted periods and hot flushes and that any others, such as palpitations, irritability, insomnia, fatigue and emotional instability, were manifestations of anxiety and depression that occurred frequently in mid-life but related only temporarily to the menopause. 'There is no evidence,' he stated, 'that this group of complaints is due to estrogen deficit or that it is alleviated by administration of estrogens.' Further, he noted, 'evidence that the dread and fear with which many women in civilized groups approach the menopause is less common in more primitive societies'.[27]

These insidious fears were perpetrated by the 'living decay' described by the American gynaecologist Robert Wilson. Menopause, he proclaimed, was a tragedy 'borne bravely by women, but . . . hardly endurable' as it reduced them all to useless 'castrates'. Redundant and obsolete, their bodies were a 'galloping catastrophe' which only oestrogen could repair and make them for their husbands 'much more pleasant to live with . . . not dull and unattractive'. Wilson published *Feminine Forever* in 1966 and it became a bestseller just as, interestingly, the women's liberation movement was getting into gear. It turns out that Wilson, according to the *New York Times*, was funded by the pharmaceutical firm Wyeth, who now claim not to know if Wilson ever worked for them but whose profits from HRT took off over the next thirty years. Wyeth placed an advert in the *Journal of the American Medical Association* in 1975 which claimed that 'almost any tranquillizer might calm her down but at her age estrogen might be what she really needs'. The book and the adverts provided a powerful push to the medico-cultural idea of the menopause as a disease and now one with an effective 'cure', but at a cost. Wilson's son has been reported as saying that his mother, who had taken HRT, had died of breast cancer in 1988 and that she kept her illness secret to protect her husband's reputation.[28]

Medical apologists for Wilson's book praise its 'message of hope' even if it is written in a 'style of passionate, sometimes paranoid journalism', a book of 'more heart than science but . . . not a bad book at all'. Wilson's 'hyperbole', astonishingly, is even described as 'prophetic and modest to the point of understating the case', despite his being shunned and vilified by his contemporaries for his outrageous plea for long-term oestrogen therapy 'to the grave'. He still had his supporters in the late 1980s when gynaecologists John Studd and Malcolm Whitehead edited *The Menopause* (1988), including an introduction from Robert Greenblatt, another 'medical prophet', who had written the preface to *Feminine Forever*. Studd and Whitehead, with their hideously inappropriate, crusading language of prophets and wars, argued that there was now

little serious controversy about the devastating effects of oestrogen deficiency or the beneficial effects of hormone replacement therapy in post-menopausal women. Pockets of resistance remain, more spiritual than medical, but fundamentally the news concerning heart attacks, strokes and

carcinoma of the uterus is good. Some minor skirmishes
regarding the dose and the route of oestrogens, and the correct progestogens for the prevention of endometrial
pathology remain, but essentially the battle has been fought
and won.[29]

Others were not so triumphantly sanguine. Barbara and
Gideon Seaman, authors of *Women and the Crisis in Sex Hormones*
(1978), gave their Christian viewpoint against interference in
nature. The chapter on menopause is entitled 'ERT: Promise
her anything, but give her . . . Cancer'. Objecting to the
casual use of hormones since the 1940s, they claimed that
'millions upon millions of American women have faithfully
swallowed sex hormones, prescribed by their physicians', and
in a fit of wishful thinking they argue that women don't
want their natural functions 'potently modified' any more.
Hot flushes should be treated with 'wholesome remedies',
such as ginseng, vitamins and minerals, and good nutrition,
not with 'a cancer-and-cholesterol pill'. Women didn't need
to make guinea pigs of themselves and they had no obligation
to support the pharmaceutical industry, which was unrelenting in pushing its hormone preparations. Some of the
early corporate adverts are startlingly manipulative in hind-
sight – one shows a woman hopelessly clutching Delta airline
tickets with her husband standing behind her, glaring at his
watch. 'Bon Voyage?', says the copy. 'Suddenly she'd rather
not go. She's waited thirty years for this trip. Now she just
doesn't have the "bounce". She has headaches, hot flashes,
and she feels tired and nervous all the time. And for no
reason at all she cries.' Yet another, cruelly suggestive, advertised its pills 'for the menopausal symptoms that bother him
most'.[30]

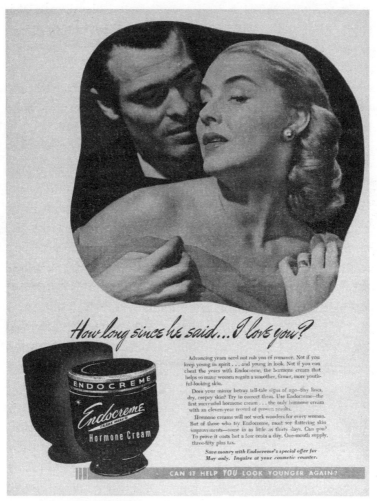

A 1940s advert sums up the message to menopausal women: just a few cents a day and a man might, possibly, still want you (not, as today, because you're worth it, but because you're cheap).

A potent mix of anthropology, religion, medical knowledge and 'nature's laws' held a woman in her alleged proper place. Rather than this being a conscious and overwhelmingly patriarchal conspiracy, many physicians truly believed in and did not see the need to question traditionally held assumptions about the nature and workings of the female sex. Their science, even as it attempted to palliate symptoms, could easily be fitted to punitive and moralistic cultural ideals and political and economic ends, even as society was slowly moving on. One physician, writing at the very end of the nineteenth century, had already begun worrying that men seemed 'afraid of offending' women and revealed a gulf between science and everyday life by claiming that 'the true differences between men and women have never been pointed out, except in medical publications'.[31] As a consequence, the medical profession had become parasitically protective, expending a great deal of energy and wordage in arguing its case from behind the parapet of the disinterested professional. Physicians were held in a cleft stick – from all the obviously hostile, misogynistic rhetoric there emerged, too, the benevolent humanity that attempted to palliate the adversities that some women undoubtedly went through as they negotiated their menopause. What was needed was discernment, an understanding of who required what treatment, if any, and an acknowledgement of the individual experience of menopause.

7

A QUESTION OF 'MALE MENOPAUSE'

> Help me! help me! now I call
> To my pretty witchcrafts all;
> Old I am, and cannot do
> That I was accustomed to . . .
>
> Find that medicine, if you can,
> For your dry, decrepit man
> Who would feign his strength renew,
>   were it but to pleasure you.

From 'To His Mistresses' in *Hesperides: or The Works both Humane and Divine of Robert Herrick Esq.* (1648)

Impotence has always been a cause of anxiety and in the past it has provided a lucrative market for a host of flamboyant quacks, clairvoyants, mesmerizers, faith-healers and anatomical museums. Today the potential is even greater as the existence of a male menopause with a familiar and extensive list of treatable symptoms is hotly debated. The male version is said to produce depression, nervousness, flushes, sweats, insomnia, bad temper, fatigue, weight gain, lowered bone mineral density, visual spatial ability deficiencies, poor concentration, poor memory, risk factors for coronary artery disease, decreased libido and erectile dysfunction.[1] Just as the sexual lives of women are supposedly ruined by menopause, so are those of men.

Historically, all manner of diabolical means, 'spells, cabalistic words, Charmes, Characters, Images, Amulets, Ligatures, Philatures, Incantations, etc.', have been used to cure, or sometimes cause, impotence. So much that is successfully 'masculine' is, and always has been, invested in an erection. Robert Burton's *Anatomy of Melancholy*, first published in 1621, bent medicine, legend, anecdote, wit, philosophy and poetry to getting and keeping one.[2] John Wilmot, 2nd Earl of Rochester, wrote impassioned verse on impotence. *The Imperfect Enjoyment* is a lover's lament, cursing the dart which has failed to please the object of his desire:

> Stiffly resolved, 'twould carelessly invade
> Woman or man, nor aught its fury stayed:
> Where'er it pierced, a cunt it found or made –
> Now languid lies in this unhappy hour,
> Shrunk up and sapless, like a withered flower.

Rochester died a young man at only thirty-three, but he composed lines on impotence in old age too, in *A Song of a Young Lady to her Ancient Lover*:

> Thy nobler part, which but to name
> In our sex would be counted shame,
> By age's frozen grasp possessed

From his ice shall be released,

And, soothed by my reviving hand,

In former warmth and vigour stand.

The young woman, whilst abashed at calling a spade a spade, believes that she can restore her elderly lover's erection, that his incapacity is but temporary. Impotence might be a terrible anxiety or intractable fear for many men but it hadn't yet been pathologized or brought into any medical syndrome.

By the mid nineteenth century, however, there were some physicians who obviously believed that men underwent a climacteric, or some distinct process of change akin to the female menopause, with a corresponding loss of sexual prowess. George Corfe thought that it occurred in males in what he called the sixth stage of life, from forty-nine to seventy years of age, and constituted 'Life's Great Climacteric Epoch'. He identified 'Singular and Curious Metamorphoses' that included those 'organs which have now ceased to take active part in the *rôle* of man's reproduction [these] are most liable to be the seat of . . . mal-transformation'.[3] Corfe didn't just concentrate on the loss of sexual function, he also noted an increasing brittleness of bones and their tendency to fractures: 'the most interesting, *natural* decay in man, is to be met with in the skeleton of his body'. He was describing the process of ageing, there being no one point at which a specific biological change occurs in men in middle-age. To Corfe, there may have been a male menopause that paralleled the timing of the female one, but it did not render a man worthless, ugly or barren, it did not affect his social status, and impotence was but one possible symptom of the passing of years.

Ever the repressive stoic, William Acton thought men should be men and not allow impotence to affect their state of mind. In *The Functions and Disorders of the Reproductive Organs* (1857), Acton offered cold comfort to the unhappily deprived man by suggesting that he should by all accounts expect a diminution of sexual passion. Portraying sexual arousal in later-middle and old age as a wholly unnatural state, he added a Christian admonishment that sex was an unwelcome interruption on a man's journey to spiritual perfection.[4]

Sylvanus Stall peddled a divinely organized male and female menopausal synchronicity when, aged fifty-four, he published *What a Man of Forty-Five Ought to Know* in 1901 in Britain and America. He wrote:

> if the wife is to lose her power to conceive and to bear children, it is but reasonable to expect that the natures, which had during the long years of wedded life been suited to each other as the different parts of a complex but perfect machine, should now find, both in the husband and in the wife such mutual physical changes as should continue to harmonise their lives during the remainder of their days.

Extolling the ideal of sexual, or non-sexual, harmony in marriage, he warned that if things were to 'wither' then all other harmonious relations would too.

> It is usually at the age of fifty or sixty that the generative function becomes weakened. It is at this period that man, elevated to the sacred character of paternity, and proud of his virile power, begins to notice the power decreased, and does so almost with a feeling of indignation. The first step towards

feebleness announces to him, unmistakeably, that he is no longer the man he was.

The thought of a sexually demanding, post-menopausal woman with an unrestrained sensuality, paired with an unmanned husband was an unspoken, unthinkable possibility, yet it lurked just beneath the surface of acceptable popular medical advice and the 'perfect machine' of marriage. Men were not described as menopausal castrates; that would have been too near the bone. What could be done to help restore the older, flagging male whose 'feebleness . . . is in part due to the diminution of the function of the testicles'? Charles-Édouard Brown-Séquard had been experimenting on a rejuvenating elixir since the 1850s. Based on his research into hormones he prepared a substance that he self-administered with a hypodermic and which, he said, gave him greater strength, vigour, mental activity and had 'increased the arc of his urine'. In 1889, when he was in his seventies, he wrote several letters to the Society of Biology in Paris showing, he said, 'the remarkable effects produced on myself by subcutaneous injection of a liquid obtained by the maceration on a mortar of the testicle of a dog or of a guineapig to which one has added a little water'. Brown-Séquard's experiments were much debated by the medical profession in Britain and America, and by the public, most of whom were said to be, at the very least, unsettled by his work. The *BMJ* published an article, 'The pentacle of rejuvenescence', which likened his ideas to 'the wild imaginings of medieval philosophers in search of an elixir vitae'. Greeted with a degree of contempt, Brown-Séquard replied with an attack on 'medicasters and charlatans' who exploited and distorted both his research and the human desire for such an elixir. Despite the furore, not to mention the risks of infection and possible side-effects of the experiments, a Dr Borrell later gave a paper to the Society of Biology saying that

> Within weeks, testicular extract was being given to patients with every kind of illness. Within two years, many physicians thought that not only the testes, but every organ of the body possessed some active principle which might be of immediate therapeutical value [and the] hope of physicians from Cleveland to Bucharest.

Although Brown-Séquard's sensational extracts had attracted a good deal of derision, the idea of 'internal secretions' had been brought into a very public arena.[5] Men suffering a lack of vigour could also try the allegedly rejuvenating monkey-gland operation, devised and carried out by a Parisian surgeon, Serge Voronoff. By the mid-1920s Voronoff had grafted the testicular tissue of chimpanzees or baboons into ageing male humans over 1000 times. He owned, conveniently and profitably, a monkey farm on the Italian Riviera. His youth-restoring operation made an appearance in Arthur Conan Doyle's Sherlock Holmes tale *The Adventure of the Creeping Man*, wherein a 61-year-old physiologist, Professor Presbury, self-administers injections of monkey serum in the weeks prior to his marriage to a much younger woman. The misguided and unfortunate professor regains his youthful vigour but is discovered dexterously swinging, simian-like, from the branches of a tree in his garden. Disgust and fear of degenerate ape-like humanity was a familiar anxiety often aired in Victorian newspaper exposés of the rising 'underclass'. Holmes's warning remark that 'When one tries to rise above Nature, one is liable to fall below it' touches on the

anxieties about society and national fitness as well as the contemporary friction between religion and science. Distorting
nature might be morally wrong or socially dangerous and
heaven only knew what the consequences might be.

Despite the disquiet the research continued and men
queued up for treatments. Having established that the physical and behavioural characteristics of sex were controlled by
testicular and ovarian hormones, Eugen Steinach attempted
to help with men's sexual difficulties by manipulating their
'glands'.[6] Transplanting ovaries into male guinea pigs, he
recorded that they displayed what he considered to be more
'feminine' behaviours and characteristics and went on to
'treat' homosexuality by removing a testicle and replacing it
with one from a heterosexual donor. His first subject, a
thirty-year-old man, allegedly began to have heterosexual
dreams, to visit a female prostitute and to develop a more
masculine body. Within months he was married and claiming
to be 'disgusted to think of a time when I felt that other passion'. We should remember that this was also a time when
that 'other passion' had been only very recently in the dock,
and had seen Oscar Wilde pilloried and destroyed. Another of
Steinach's patients was the poet W. B. Yeats, whose work had
suffered during his late sixties but who found that being
'Steinached', having a vasectomy, had greatly revived his creative power. It revived his sexual desire, too, which he hoped
and believed would 'in all likelihood' last him until he died.
Yeats thought that if he repressed his newly awoken libido
'for any long period [he] would break down under the strain
as did the great Ruskin'. The operation took place in London
in the spring of 1934, and in September of that year he began
a relationship with the young actress and poet Margot
Ruddock, who was twenty-seven years old to his sixty-nine.[7]

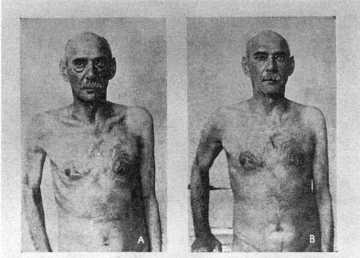

(a) SEVENTY YEAR OLD PATIENT BEFORE THE STEINACH OPERATION
(b) TWO MONTHS AFTER THE STEINACH OPERATION
(*Ufa Steinach-Film*)

Before and after photographs of a seventy-year-old man who has been 'Steinached'.

In 1910 the nerve physician Kurt Mendel tentatively extended the controversial idea of male menopause. It was accepted by some as a valid medical entity from a psychiatric point of view. Others, including Krafft-Ebing, stoutly denied its existence, saying that 'to establish a menopause for the masculine sex, and to particularize the psychoses which are attached to this age (fifty to sixty years) does not seem to me admissible from either the biologic or the clinical point of view'. The 'masculine menopause' was not a fact: 'It appears to be rather the result of the imagination of the writers who have described it.'

It was a divisive question. Marañón boldly asserted the reality *'of the critical age in the male'* as a 'stage of organic evolution, perfectly characterized, anatomically and physiologically, in whose centre the extinction of active genital life stands out prominently'. The 'line described by the human organism from birth to death is not suddenly broken into abrupt descents, like steps,' he wrote, 'it is rather a smooth, curved line divided into distinct sectors whose limits are not precise'.[8] Would that the female menopause had been seen as such a 'perfect' characterization and part of a smooth curve of growth.

Male menopause is diffuse, Marañón claimed, and 'testicular insufficiency', the 'genital extinction' and alleged central part of the masculine climacteric, occurs much more slowly and much later than does 'ovarian insufficiency' in women. Even in cases where a man 'is unable to perform the sexual act perhaps because of lack of power in the external genital apparatus, difficulty in erection, the internal testicular secretion may not be deficient', even into their nineties and older. Quaintly coy, he noted that 'doctors in asylums for the aged have observed that the principal occupation of the patients is discussion of the love question'. External contributing factors to the male menopause were listed as syphilis, alcoholic or nicotine intoxication, emotional excesses and overfatigue, 'all of which explains the intensity of, and the greater proportion of, insanity as manifested in men'.

Marañón took the condition very seriously, citing examples of 'sufferers', cases such as that of

G. C. Man fifty-nine years old; very rheumatic; always strong; active and prolonged sexual life. In this age he began to suffer from nervous disturbances with tendency to melancholia, digestive disturbances and flatulence and circulatory troubles, chiefly hypertension. These symptoms, together with a marked increase in weight – abdominal especially – I interpreted as the consequence of the masculine climacteric.

Finally, he suffered, particularly on the days he worked hard, from *violent attacks of pain which . . . at once extended over the whole head.* He had learned by himself to relieve these attacks with hot local applications [original emphasis].

Another, an actor aged fifty-five with severe arthritis and 'neuropathic antecedents', had suffered for two years from 'intense nervous phenomena, with a tendency to melancholy, intense flatulence, persistent increase in weight, localized fat on the abdomen, and various other climacteric manifestations'. One of the symptoms of which he *'complained the most was a painful restlessness in both legs, which forced him to move them continuously* whether sitting or standing, and which disturbed his performance on the stage'. A. de G., a 59-year-old artist and 'old syphilitic . . . with a very active sex life', came to Marañón with circulatory problems, dizziness, insomnia and a *'diminution of sexual power* coincident with such an increase in the *size of the abdomen* that he required new clothing'. He also had sudden *'difficult and prolonged . . . great accumulation of gas'*, together with respiratory difficulty, 'loss of emotional control' and a 'psychic state of jealousy toward younger men in his profession', all very characteristic, thought his doctor, 'of male psychology in this age' [original emphasis]. Farting, nerves, melancholy and a sense of diminution could be added to Marañón's swelling list of 'symptoms'.

Homosexual 'inversion' was rarer, he thought, than lesbianism, though a tendency to submission could be discerned, even if 'outside the home no normal man is the slave of the woman'. Men had confessed to him that 'they were now moved emotionally by things to which they were formerly indifferent' but, of course, they suffered 'with rather less intensity than in woman'. Rheumatism, diabetes, asthma, weight loss, urinary and cutaneous problems, impatience, neurasthenia, an 'evolution toward conservatism' and emotional instability were common complaints but sexual melancholy, if it struck, was especially hard if men had been Don Juans in their prime. Marañón illustrated this affliction with an extract from a novel by E. Monfort, *La belle-enfant ou l'amour a 40 ans* (1918). The hero is undone:

> Forty years! He was forty years old! His age was written in every bit of him, in the flabbiness of his face, in the heaviness of his body, while his heart, not aged, but still young, beat as though it were at its twenty-fifth year. Forty years! Pleasure was ended, no longer could he interest women. Having reached the end of youth, having passed the time of love, what pleasure in life now remained to him? The obsession of the lost paradise, the thought of things past, the ever present memory of the enchanted country where he had once been and whither he can never more return! All is lost at this age . . . He beheld himself in a mirror. The image was terrible. Impossible to retain the least illusion that he was the same being. He saw the whole disagreeable transformation, his wrinkles, the crow's feet they had made in his cheeks, the flabbiness of his skin, his thick neck. He was withered, worn out. He was old. Fifteen years before he had seen a man of about this age go out of the house and he now recalled exactly the impression which he had produced, the painful sense of physical ruin, a pot-bellied being in a shirt, dishevelled, his eyes swollen, his legs hairy. The spectacle had been grotesque and lamentable. And now he himself was like that man.

'The hero was inconsolable; stronger men, less effeminate characters . . . suffer in only a transient way . . . Maturity of spirit, more complete possession of themselves, intellectual and moral benefit compensate them for the physical loss.' He is too womanly, obviously, and feels deeply, and rightly, his loss of sexual power. But sexual uselessness and social castration were not the inevitability for men that they were for women. Marañón maintained he might yet find success as his 'heart does not acquire full capacity for love and for every delicate or passionate sentiment until between the fortieth and fiftieth years', when he will be 'more seductive than at any other time'. His economic and social position was stronger too, for a man's social status, unlike a woman's, had a sexual value. Menopause was not the gateway to death for a man.

The first detailed popular exposition of the male menopause, in Stall's book *What a Man of Forty-Five Ought to Know*, was 'well-received in both medical and religious circles' and contained no fewer than eighteen chapters on what men might expect in mid-life, including enlargement of the prostate, late marriage, the change of life in women, how to cope with the 'mental manifestations', the 'preservation of virility' and the many compensations it apparently heralded. That at least some of the problems were sexual was subtly hinted at by a review in the *Journal of Dermatology*: 'A reliable and instructive guide in sexual matters and yet pure and chaste in style.' The *Medical World* noted that 'These cases are often very troublesome to the physician. It would be well to have this book handy to lend to such patients . . . to manage his patient and help the patient. This book will do much good. There has been a need for just such a work.'[9] A companion volume, E. F. Angell Drake's *What a Woman of Forty-Five Ought to Know* (1902), informed a wife that her husband, like her, would 'come to a time of life when he has not quite the mental and physical poise he once had'. Patience, Drake declared, 'is as much a cardinal virtue in the wife towards her husband, at this time, as in

the husband towards the wife' men, who had been so patient
with their irrational and difficult wives, would now require the
reciprocal understanding of these women. Psychological and
physiological difficulties of mid-life – disappointment, perhaps – and physical signs of ageing, which might include
impotence, were obviously bringing some men to the physician's door. A male menopause provided a blanket diagnosis in
the face of all these amorphous complaints, giving both doctor
and patient something to hang on to and even something to
do, with a new regime or even a hormone or two.

In America, doctors E. B. Lowry and R. J. Lambert argued
that the male menopause could affect men at about fifty-
five years of age. In their book *Himself: Talks with Men Concerning
Themselves* (Chicago, 1912), they were, however, just as vague
about possible symptoms, suggesting that a man of these
years might have

> a few months during which he experiences a condition of
> anxiety and unrest; he does not seem able to accomplish his
> desires; he feels generally weak, and a tendency to weeping
> becomes manifest . . . headache, heart palpitation, sleepless-
> ness, vertigo, mental depression, failure of memory and
> attention, and impairment of sexual power and desire. As a
> rule, this period does not last more than a year and then the
> man may apparently resume his accustomed vigour. Seldom
> is the disturbance attributed to its proper cause.

This didn't mean, they assured their readers, that a man
should 'quietly wait the end' like a washed-up woman.
Unlike her, he is so much more than a baby-maker; some of
his best work can be done 'after this period of life', and some
of his best experiences were yet to come.

The sexual mythology that surrounded the menopause had encouraged the idea that sex was desired and desirable in youth alone, but many of the poignant letters received by Marie Stopes put this one to bed. A clergyman wrote to her in great distress, saying:

> I am fifty-one years of age, married and have a boy aged seventeen and a girl of twenty-two years of age. Both are sound in every way – mentally and physically. Lately, i.e. during the last six months, I have been unable to achieve an erection – or at all events a very fleeting one. So fleeting that I am unable to penetrate. My wife is naturally disappointed though she is, if anything, undersexed. She has accused me of infidelity, but I have succeeded in persuading her that I am not guilty *only* impotent. She naturally asks '*Why?*'[10]

Stopes reassured him that he was passing through the change of life, that in women it was simply the cessation of menstrual flow, an incident in the longer climacteric period which was complemented in men by a 'temporary impotence or cessation of active sex capacity'. In healthy men, she said, it was a brief interlude lasting but a few months or a year or two.

In her massively popular book *Change of Life in Men and Women* (London, 1936), Stopes made it plain that she accepted the idea of male menopause but, as much as she wanted to 'demolish the widespread bogey-belief' of the risks of the female menopause, she didn't want to turn the tables on men. There was, she said, a singular silence about the corresponding 'crisis' in men, which meant to her only that they passed through it easily and fearlessly, not that it didn't actually exist. She thought that the 'blindness of many members

of the medical profession to the existence of a male climacteric is so extraordinary it seems wilful'. There were only
three pages on 'The male critical age' in surgeon Kenneth
Walker's book *Sex Difficulties in the Male* (London, 1934), for
instance, and Leonard Williams, in *Middle Age and Old Age*
(London, 1925), 'bounded by inborn ideas of masculine dom-
ination', argued that if it was 'to be admitted that there is
ever such a thing as a male climacteric, it must be held to
refer to men with a strong homosexual tendency, and to
them only'. Stopes retaliated, waspishly, that this may have
been what male doctors wanted to believe, but it was not
true. She thought it was the manly, strongly sexed type who
suffered most. For example, the distraught clergyman who,
as a boy, had been instructed in masturbation by an older
boy and had continued with it till he married, who described
himself as strong, healthy, lean and hard, nearly six feet tall,
with a forty-inch chest and weighing 12 st. 10 lbs, a man who
had played first-class rugby football for years, and played forward for his county. Physically he considered himself no
weakling except in this one sensitive area of his otherwise
successful and fulfilled life. Until he became impotent his
marriage had been happy, but:

Now it is in danger of being wrecked. Sometimes I ejaculate
as soon as I touch my wife and that ends all effort. As a result
of all this failure I feel 'a worm and no man', feel depressed
and desperate. My work suffers and, obsessed with this feeling of hopelessness, I feel desperate – at the end of my
tether . . . What can I do? I *want* to do my duty to my wife –
we love one another as we have always done, and I hope
shall continue to do so. Here we have no *experienced* doctor
whom I could consult. They are all too young and would

laugh at me. I've heard them do it to others similarly situated. Could you help? As a clergyman – of very limited
means – my position is a very delicate one, as you can well
understand. I have tried various things, e.g. 'D-----s,' which
I dare say are useless. But when one is in my mental state one
will try *anything* in the desperate hope that it will accomplish
what is claimed of it. I have been greatly tempted to put an
end to it all and to send myself to that country where 'they
neither marry nor are given in marriage.' In fact a few days
before your excellent book came into my hands I got out
my old army revolver, but thought I ought to see my boy
launched on his career before I finish mine . . . Please help
me!

The age at which impotence might occur was thought to
vary enormously, as did the desire of the wives of these men.
One correspondent, a man of seventy-five, had found himself
'somewhat failing, not competent to really satisfy my wife of
sixty-eight years as she should be satisfied'. And a letter from
a 49-year-old man confided that,

to be frank, some six weeks ago whilst attempting with my
wife my marital duties as a husband, I failed, and the fact of
that so got upon my mind I seem ever since to live in a state
of terror of being unable to accomplish the act that I *do fail*,
and this despite a virile erection (pardon me) and then
'falling' immediately.

He wrote to Stopes, almost prostrate with grief, for his home
life was in a state of chaos and his wife believed he had been
unfaithful to her. Stopes sympathized with his terrible distress and reasoned that, even though it seemed cruel to

deflate male conceit and their desire to dominate, it was less cruel to recognize openly and generally make this problem known so that lives and marriages would not continue to be wrecked through ignorance. 'How little men know about men!' she exclaimed. 'In their freest, coarsest gossip among themselves men rarely talk of this thing,' and the 'cock-sure' ones could even turn nastily on their wives and blame them.[11]

That, or they could turn to the 'quack drug stores' which specialized in commercial products professing to restore virility. Thyroid extract was easy to obtain and known to 'work wonders in the climacteric man, as it does in climacteric women' even if it was largely unregulated and thought to be potentially dangerous. '*On no account*,' insisted Stopes, should these thyroid, testicular and prostatic extracts be injected, nor should men take dried tablets, just 'freshly prepared gelatine-coated extracts from a scientific laboratory' and never over the counter from a high street chemist's shop. These preparations were not a cure, she counselled, and might have to be taken daily in small doses for several months, possibly even years, to have any effect at all.

Stopes also recommended letting one's house and travelling, varying the weekends by hiking, and drinking beer – though certainly not for women. But by far the most effective remedy for impotence would have to be electricity, despite the lack of agreement as to the best way in which it might be applied. Stopes suggests that the special applicator should be inserted very gently into the rectum and should not be moved about, but just held still while the current runs and then removed. This must be preferable to the disgrace of finding oneself in court should the 'happy husband and father' with an 'unbalanced enlargement of the

local glandular tissue of the prostate' take up, in consequence, a 'sudden sex-interest in young girls, petting and
fondling them'. Should this disorder happen, though, a wise
and self-respecting wife should not take personal offence, but
should see that the affair is hushed up, and that proper medical attention is given to her suffering husband.[12]

Despite some acceptance of the phenomenon of male
menopause it was a concept with a dubious history still
viewed with some suspicion in the 1920s and 30s. It lacked the
historical context of the female variety. There was no specialization comparable with gynaecology and the male sex
hormone market did not take off in the same headlong way
as did HRT for women. Hormonal treatment for impotent
men was common in Germany by the late 1930s but Western
orthodox medicine was still largely disputing its worth,
believing instead that the condition was more psychological
than physiological, even though, curiously, depression and
schizophrenia were treated with these preparations. The first
active preparation of male hormone was produced in 1927
from the lipid fraction of bull's testis. Androsterone was isolated in 1931 and synthesized in 1934, and a year later
crystalline testosterone was prepared.[13] In 1931 the pharmaceutical company Organon carried out small-scale trials of
Hombreol in the US, consulting with the sceptical psychiatrists. They advertised in the *Lancet* with the line, 'A man aged
60 complained of impotence . . . After a preliminary course of
injections . . . potency was regained [and] apart from the
maintenance of sexual function, the most obvious effects
have been the new growth of hair and an increase in virility.'
In 1935 testosterone was isolated and identified and a cheap
synthetic preparation became available. Organon began
manufacturing Testosteron two years later. Their research

suggested to them that the new male sex hormone preparations would actually affect a whole series of symptoms of old age in men, not only sexual functions. They might also 'bring about favourable effects in a psychological sense' – real wonder drugs of rejuvenation.[14]

But there was criticism from within the ranks. In 1939 the *Journal of the American Medical Association* carried an article by the Council on Pharmacy and Chemistry which slammed what it called extravagant and grossly exaggerated claims being made for male sex hormones, claims which were appearing, worryingly, in both medical journals and the public newspapers and magazines. Wildly potent promises of eternal manhood were blasted as 'immature' and 'should be disregarded'. All very sensible until you compare their attitude with their silence on the concurrent universal demands for women to be eternally 'feminine', attractive, sexually viable and available.

In 1944, following more advances in endocrinology, the *Journal of the American Medical Association* published what was to be an influential paper by Heller and Myers, 'The male climacteric, its symptomatology, diagnosis and treatment'.[15] It described and detailed the 'symptomatology, diagnosis and treatment' of a discrete medical condition which began to be spoken and written of as the 'andropause' or 'viropause'. It was associated almost entirely with a decline in testosterone levels. The argument was that low levels of testosterone could be reversed by hormone replacement therapy but not by placebo, strongly indicating a physiological 'problem', treatable with the help of the pharmaceutical companies.

The American biologist Alfred Kinsey's 1948 bestseller, *Sexual Behavior in the Human Male*, found no evidence of a mid-life male climacteric. According to his research, male sexual activity peaked in the teens and began a slow, life-long decline, with no sudden lack of vigour in the fifties. At age sixty 5 per cent were sexually inactive, at seventy 30 per cent, 'yet even in old age impotence was often attributed more to psychological than physiological causes'. Sex therapy was taking off. In 1952 the American Psychiatric Association's *Diagnostic and Statistical Manual of Mental Disorders* had listed impotence as psychologically based. The research partners, gynaecologist William Masters and psychologist Virginia Johnson, who published *Human Sexual Response* in 1966, pinpointed long-term negative thinking, including depression, anger, fear and boredom, as the main causes of sexual decline in men. Like Kinsey they reported that 'consistency of active sexual expression' from middle-age on was a key factor. They claimed that men over fifty could be trained out of 'secondarily acquired impotence', so virility could be reconstituted or restimulated. Monotony, fatigue and illness all played a part in male anxiety, as well as the 'heavy burden of male responsibility in sexual intercourse'.[16]

A clamour began for medical intervention and immediate results and, of course, sparked off huge commercial interest. In the 1970s and 80s men were still being recommended the vacuum devices and herbs that their Victorian fathers and grandfathers had used, but new remedies were appearing on the market too. Injections of vasodilating substances costing up to $2400 a year, risky bypass surgery of penile arteries and implants were being offered. The implants of silicone rods came in three models: the Malleable 600 Penile Prosthesis, consisting of two silicone rubber rods which could be bent for comfort or straightened for penetration; the Dynaflex Penile Prosthesis, with two little fluid-filled cylinders that inflated when squeezed; and the 700 Ultrex Inflatable Penile Prosthesis, which had a tiny reservoir and pump hidden in the scrotum. Advertisements for these aids had wives rapturously reporting that their husbands 'were more relaxed and confident'. An implant operation could set you back up to $9000, yet within a decade 250,000 to 300,000 procedures had been undertaken, and by 1995 American men were spending $6-7 million a year on their virility.[17]

The Pfizer pharmaceutical company, which produced sildenafil citrate, or Viagra (the name was coined from the words 'vigour' and 'niagara'), said it had stumbled across its potential as a sex drug during other research in the late 1980s. It began human testing in 1990 and eight years later Viagra became the first oral medication approved by the United States Food and Drug Administration to treat 'erectile dysfunction'. This term was replacing 'impotence' and shifting the emphasis from a character flaw to a vascular problem, giving the impression that it was a condition which could be 'cured'; all this was backed by the corporate funding of research into sexual dysfunction. During the 1990s an American sex survey found that sexual inactivity jumped in men over sixty, though Masters and Johnson had speculated that only about 5 per cent of men over sixty experienced a climacteric life change, still begging the question of whether 'male menopause' was a physiological or psychological entity, and whether it was directed or enhanced by medico-cultural trends.[18]

Much is known about the supply of Viagra but little about the demand for it, nor whether it increases male anxiety or relieves it. Pfizer stock rose 150 per cent in 1998 when the drug was approved, and sales of Viagra topped $1 billion in 1999, giving a profit margin of 90 per cent as it became the fastest-selling pharmaceutical in history. It is debatable whether this was a hitherto hidden market or one that was created by a sophisticated campaign to convince men they needed it for their intractable 'medical condition'. Researchers who published an oft-cited article in the *Journal of the American Medical Association* in 1999, stating that 43 per cent of women and 31 per cent of men had a 'sexual dysfunction' (whatever that is) that posed an 'important public health concern', had failed to disclose their links to Pfizer. Initially Pfizer had marketed the drug at 'respectable' middle-aged and elderly married men, even seeking the tacit support of churches and the Vatican. But when sales plateaued in 2000 the focus shifted to the baby boomers, though half the men who tried it did not renew their prescriptions. Deaths in the first year were attributed to pre-existing conditions but side-effects in healthy men were acknowledged, including a flushed face, headaches and blueish vision. Other, competing drugs began to appear, such as Cialis, Icos and Levitra, and Pfizer started to concentrate on the potentially very lucrative female market of sexual dysfunction. All this is greatly aided by direct-to-consumer advertising and the remarkably persistent notion of romance even though the drugs are all about blood flow.

In 2000 the *British Medical Journal* was still asking whether the male menopause actually existed or not, though most medical authorities now believe that it is a myth and that any changes presented are more psychological than physiological.[19] The novelist John Fowles recorded in his journal in November 1988, when he was aged sixty-two, that he was impotent, had seen a doctor and had been told that his testosterone count was low. He and his wife, Elizabeth, were 'sent away to think it over'. She thought they 'should leave it alone' and was alarmed by the thought of 'having sex'; he thought that if he did nothing 'it will cause no harm . . . though in some way (some lingering folk-belief, perhaps) I feel it must, psychologically'. Fowles regarded his impotence as a 'castration' which in effect separated him 'from the rest of humankind, or their common experience . . . I haven't really absorbed its implications as yet'. In March the following year Fowles despairingly confides that 'Eliz "doesn't know who she is" anymore, has lost identity. I feel the same.'[20] Being at a loss is no surprise as many of the reported 'symptoms' of the male menopause mirror the exhaustive lists for the female menopause.

There is no 'point of reference' for men as there is for women with their last period, so those who argue for the male menopause concentrate on the levels of testosterone in the blood which allow for sexual functioning, by which they mean a sustainable erection. The argument is that, as oestrogen levels decline in women as they age, so do testosterone levels decrease as men get older, often with exaggerated falls in the evening hours. Levels of testosterone which support a sustainable erection are found in 99 per cent of healthy men aged between twenty and forty. Levels below this occur in 20 per cent of men aged between sixty and eighty and in 33 per cent aged over eighty.[21] Genetics plays a role but other risk factors for early or dramatic falls in testosterone are a history of inflammation of, or trauma to, the testes, obesity, diabetes and excess alcohol intake; the influence of physical and psychological stress is still a matter for debate.

To the 'Body and Gut' mind of orthodox medicine, the fact that both a decline in sexual interest and potency and a fall in testosterone levels occur with ageing suggests that sexual behaviour is largely dependent on testosterone levels.

Some doctors believe that the debate is unnecessary as, whether you call it the male menopause or not, men with age-related decline in sexual interest and functionality can be 'helped by their physician' and drugs, apparently solving the problem.[22] Some argue that men *need* andrologists to help them through problems with 'health, sexual and marital issues' and that they have not been as well served as women have by gynaecologists, nor are they able to talk to their GPs or friends in an open and fearless manner. Perhaps, though, what they don't need is to be patronized by professionals who accuse them of 'embarrassed incomprehension' and of having 'trouble telling the truth about their sex lives but . . . still need our help'. Help that is available 'in the form of testosterone'.[23]

The pharmaceutical companies who need to exploit the new market – and, as we're on the subject, the higher inci-dences of prostate cancer – have devised snappy little acronyms to promote their research and products, such as ADAM – Androgen Decline in the Ageing Male, or PEDAM – the Partial Endocrine Deficiency in the Adult Male. The latter, whilst not quite so catchy, at least does not include the possi-bly off-putting words 'ageing' and 'decline'. But older men given testosterone supplements (orally, or by injection, patches or implants) which raised their levels to those of a twenty-year-old man experienced no beneficial effects on bone mineral density or muscle strength, though they did become leaner. An article in the *Lancet* in 2007 on 'sexual dys-function in men and women with endocrine disorders' argued that the decline in testosterone production in ageing men is not associated with precise sexual symptoms, and that taking the hormone does not do much for their potency either. Up to 80 per cent of cases of erectile dysfunction are thought to stem from illnesses such as diabetes, cardiovascular disease, neurological disorders (such as multiple sclerosis or spinal injuries), prostate surgery and trauma. And the side-effects of supplementation are sufficient to raise the alarm, including, as they do, a possible increase in heart attacks, weight gain, insomnia and the problem with arguably the greatest impact: the stimulated growth of a small undiagnosed prostate cancer.

Most doctors or andrologists are against the idea of testosterone replacement therapy, which has had 'very, very few scientific trials to support its use', because of the cancer risk. Knowing that an effective treatment of advanced prostate cancer is to remove testosterone by drug treatment or surgery, it would seem absurd to be delivering it almost blindly.[24] It is not too reductive or crude to look back several decades and wonder at the lack of such opposition to drug treatment for the female menopause.

Those who argue against the idea of a male menopause say that change is gradual and that any apparent symptoms cannot be definitely or confidently laid at the door of testosterone deficiency. The symptoms could just as well be ascribed to other endocrine changes associated with getting older and with changes in a man's life circumstances, personality or environment – just as in the female menopause. Professor Kirkwood states emphatically that, 'in spite of claims to the contrary, there is no such thing as a male menopause', and argues that while men lose fertility due to age changes in their testes and may find it increasingly difficult to get and maintain an erection, they do not experience a specific shutdown of reproductive function. And whilst men may have a gradual decrease in testosterone they do not invariably experience it as women do, whose oestrogen levels will always decline during the menopausal transition. Treatments for the many alleged symptoms of female menopause have undoubtedly fed into the recent and increasing interest in a possible, and possibly very lucrative, male equivalent. If traditional notions of masculinity are being exploited by drug companies and some doctors it is also true that men have historically had a voice; they have not been dismissed or vilified in the same way as menopausal women. Perhaps after centuries of denigration of the female menopause men are reluctant to have one of their own.

8

FINDING A VOICE

God! Oh make it stop,
This change!
Don't take the blood out of my body!
. . .
Flutter of fear in the nerves
Where before the assurance chuckled!
Along the nerves, a low throbbing,
A slow, heavy patter of lessening vibration
Lowered to pain.

Rosy best of the blood gone out of my body!
Deserter!
. . .
Death! Death! Take me with you to spare
      me this last!

                    D. H. Lawrence, 'Change of Life'

Blood, being and the soul were not just the preserve of
earthy, florid and avowedly masculine poets whose view of
menopause was that even death might be the preferable

option. Medicine, too, had long ago appropriated cultural meaning for its own and reinforced its influence over what constituted essential femaleness. During the twentieth century, however, women began to assert their own version of menopause and what it meant to them. They must refuse, wrote Marie Stopes, 'to be bullied into miserable ill-health by the primitive, dominating male, whose open contempt for women's whole existence save as a female breeding animal, colours his thoughts and even his medical writings'.[1] The feminist and socialist reformer Stella Browne, who had her menopause sometime during the 1920s or early 30s, discussed the subject in many of the talks on health issues she gave to women's groups, constantly emphasizing the need for women to freely speak out about their own experiences. In a paper she gave to the British Society for the Study of Sex Psychology in 1915, 'The sexual variety and variability among women and their bearing upon social reconstruction', she argued that 'in the social order for which some of us hope and work, provision will have to be made for women's periodic changes; menstruation and the menopause, must be recognised and "allowed for".' Browne was a committed campaigner; she had participated in the famous Freewoman debate of 1912 on chastity and sexual desire in women, corresponded with Havelock Ellis from 1914 until his death in 1938, was a founder of the Abortion Law Reform Association in 1936, supported the Women's Social and Political Union, the Divorce Law Reform Union, the No-Conscription Fellowship, the Humanitarian League and the Federation of Progressive Societies and Individuals. She was an early member of the British Communist Party and was active in the Labour Party and the Fabian Society as well. Browne also noted that 'many experienced medical women, whose

knowledge and judgment I respect, believe that under fair
and healthy conditions, menstruation will gradually become
almost negligible', almost as though living without periods
was actually the norm.[2]

Unfortunately, these female voices of reason were still in
the minority and prone to the terrible consequences of menstruation and menopause on 'mentality and the "soul"'. So
declared Joseph Dulberg in 1920, a physician who appeared to
view women as badly behaved children rather than as intelligent beings like Stella Browne.[3] Their ignorance and
martyrdom were a source of mental as well as physical agony
and the menopause was 'looked forward to with fear and
trepidation'. Dulberg thought very many women (for few
escaped) were horribly prone to self-deception in mid-life,
leading to a great deal of avoidable 'domestic unhappiness'.
Some got very 'amative' indeed, displaying an 'intense and
insatiable desire', which often ended in divorce through her
adultery. This moral deviation caused any number of them to
scurrilously run off with the chauffeur. Dr Dulberg's
patients, we can assume, came from the wealthy and self-
indulgent middle and upper classes, the same women whose
hysteria and neurasthenia provided such good business in
the late nineteenth century.

Dulberg was of one mind with the ancients on the excess of
blood in menopausal women's bodies and 'the impurities
contained in it which, for want of being eliminated from the
body by the menstrual discharge, circulate through the blood
vessels of the skin', causing hot flushes and affecting all their
other organs as well. As relief from these symptoms he recommended warm baths, toast, and plenty of mastication and
masturbation.

'Not only do they complain,' he complained, 'they suffer

from every possible disease under the sun, from cancer to insomnia,' and he had identified so many menopausal symptoms that it would mean 'writing a book on all the diseases known to the medical profession'. Even when faced with a patient in her early forties who was spitting blood and swearing to him that she was consumptive, Dulberg asserted that she was menopausal, attributing nothing but benefit from her symptom as a way of ridding her body of the suppressed blood. But he was quite cross that she 'would not take my word for it'. 'In the end,' he notes, 'I lost sight of her, and I am bound to confess that I did not feel in the least sorry. Such cases are by no means rare.' One wonders how many women his prejudice condemned in this way.

A woman's periodic 'emotional instability' was now enshrined as medical and scientific fact, and it had mutated into an immutable cultural truth too. It was, according to Marañón, due to endocrine disturbance, and was the most characteristic 'element common to almost all menopausal women . . . *Often it is the only psychic phenomenon of the menopause* [original emphasis].'[4] Women would most likely experience psychic complications including mania, melancholia, manic-depressive states, neurasthenia, hysteria and epilepsy. The severity, timing and duration of the menopause depended on constitution, sexual history, race, class, weight, colour of hair, previous health and temperament, and the climate. A woman's symptoms were universal, encompassing the genital, circulatory, nervous, metabolic, endocrine, digestive, cutaneous and various others of her 'organs and apparatus'. Despite his apparent in-depth and comprehensive knowledge, Marañón still thought it impossible to fix on a period of duration for the menopause and found it 'hard to decide when and when not it is pathologic'. He was sure, though, that syphilis could cause it to come early. Indeed, any 'abuses of the genital function' would accelerate the menopause, including celibacy, for it 'is delayed by normal exercise of the genital organs', although he doesn't explain what 'normal' is, nor where some happy medium of sexual activity lay. Intense emotion could bring it on abruptly, and grief, such as the death of a loved one, 'especially a husband, in certain passionate women' coinciding with 'the conviction that any future love would be impossible', would most certainly do it – nature's way of killing off the widow too, perhaps. But there was always golf, that excellent remedy, which, extraordinarily, he believed would break the 'spiritual monotony of life'. Motoring was considered very beneficial too, whereas overdoing train travel could be draining. Massage was recommended, vegetarianism and hydrotherapy also, and, if all else failed, sedation.[5]

Marañón appropriated menopausal women's voices to explain their 'peculiar psychic state'. He reprinted part of a letter he had received from a 'very brilliant and observant woman who had always been well balanced'. Now, however, 'she had been seized by disturbances attributable to an early climacteric':

Why has my character changed so much? Formerly I was very calm and now a vexation or an injustice produces in me such discomposure – so strong an emotion dominates me that others can tell it by the tremor in my voice. And I especially notice what seems to be a feeling of horrible anguish – a sensation like oppression – as if my heart (to speak unscientifically) threatened to leap from its place. What worries me most is that this excess of emotionalism is not related to causes, since if I hear something sad – no matter how sad it may be – my usual calmness is not altered in the least. Why

am I fearful, if nothing threatens? My greatest diversion used
to be to walk alone to my house in the country and to be left
there alone in peace. Now, I go as before. But when I find
myself alone there I am afraid and not of anything, but
rather of myself.

To further illustrate this irritability he used the French
novelist and dramatist Octave Feuillet's comedy *La Crise*
(1854), based, he thought, on an 'excellent knowledge of
feminine psychology', there presumably being no female
writer to quote. The main character, Julia, experiencing 'the
fullness of her sexual life and therefore within the shadow
of its close', in a *cri de coeur* asks: 'What name can be given to this
moral affliction, to this discontent with myself and with those
about me which I have felt for some months?' Her sexual
state and her emotional life are as one – she describes a decid-
edly moral, not physiological, difficulty. 'My husband,' she
continues,

is, doubtless, the best of men. But nothing that he says or
does pleases me. His watch charms irritate me above everything else. Yet these charms and I have lived together in
peace for ten years. Then suddenly, one fine day, we hate
each other. My husband has the insufferable habit of jin-
gling them while he is talking – making an unbearable
clinking. At the very instant that I write these lines he is in
his room, winding his watch and making a noise with those
charms.

This best of all possible husbands is a dignified but 'thoroughly alarmed' magistrate who runs to tell the doctor
about his wife's 'obedient, but irritated' behaviour, certain

that she is sick rather than that he is a pain. The 'wise' doctor gets straight to the point: 'I have it — your wife's age.' Marañón extends his pity to the author, certain that this tale is drawn from Feuillet's intimate life, and obviously feeling a great deal of solidarity for his sadly misunderstood and mistreated sex. And in Michaelis's novel *L'Age Dangereux* yet another apparently menopausal woman laments that

> The sight of Riccardo slowly became a torture to me. With what absolute perfection he managed his knife and fork! I could have stood it if he would ever — if only once — put his elbows on the table, or bite into an apple before peeling it, or make a noise when drinking! But no: his correctness was infallible and unchangeable! . . . his mania for correctness drove me to committing every possible solecism, just to annoy him. Sometimes I purposely disarranged the books in his library.[6]

Obviously, there must have been something wrong with the women that they should be so very irritated by their men; what other reason could there possibly have been? Women, according to Marañón, had a *'tendency, unconscious perhaps, to live intensely a group of sensations which in the natural law of life, not always in harmony with instinct, should soon end* [original emphasis]'.[7] They were indiscriminate, amatory, tumultuous and easily 'launched upon evil courses' if they felt neglected. Once her husband had 'satisfied his monogamous curiosity' she might well be drawn to look for a new passion, a 'secondary or late love' and the 'rock on which the woman in the "dangerous age" so frequently stumbles'. In *La Crise* the doctor diagnoses this as 'a normal disease which may attack the best of women, as they reach the threshold of maturity. Such is the attraction of the evil fruit which Eve held for the first time in her hands. Thus the most honoured woman may sense a desire not to be resigned to death without having tasted it.'

Some women, however, might escape these irrationalities and attain a 'psychic serenity' if their 'neuroendocrine crisis does not exceed certain limits of abnormality'. One Madame de Hauville reached this point by refusing to be reminded of her youth and believing 'that maturity and old age which it initiates is the perfect moment in which one hoards and remembers. Then all the splendours of the world appear finer. The close of life is undoubtedly more beautiful than its dawn.' The '*sensation of realizing that one is ageing*' could precipitate a sexual melancholy and a loss of sexual function, not of libido which is different, but of menstruation and beauty, meaning that, although she still wants to have sex, sex doesn't want to have her. This condition, Marañón suggests, is to be especially observed in the intensely lived lives of society women and prostitutes of all kinds 'to whom sexual success is either an explicit or a subconscious means (an honest exhibition of her beauty, her elegance, her handsome clothes) and the principal end of her existence'.[8] The woman who reaches the menopause 'surrounded by her children and who has the care of her home, may consider the object of her life accomplished and accept the loss of her reproductive power in an attitude which I have called "psychic serenity"'. Again, the attitude was: be 'good' and your suffering will be less. In the indulgent upper classes, too, where 'sexual suggestion is more acute and frequent', the menopause might be more turbulent than for lower-class, occupied women. He did not think that the upper classes might have had the resources and the physicians to consult, whereas their poorer, busier sisters would have had to go without.

Dr Hélène Wolfromm connected any female psychological instability to the fear of ageing (rather than ageism), prescribing isolation and rest cures for depressed women who acted 'irrationally' by, for instance, leaving their husbands without having 'another attachment' to go to. Women were encouraged to go on special diets, swallow sedatives, take up gymnastics or golf, to use astringent lotions and to smile a good deal less. The last would seem to be an obvious consequence of all the previous strictures and recommendations. Even in the 1920s and 30s, then, a scientific version of the menopause was intimately bound up with societal rules, class and morality.

During her forties Virginia Woolf had been fascinated by the idea of the menopause, the 'turn of life', and troubled by her doctors' advice that she should not have children. On Tuesday 24 November 1936, when she was fifty-four years old, Woolf recorded in her diary that she was glad to be dining with her friend Helen Anrep so that

> I shan't be alone, alone I fall into those trances, comas, which are I suppose t. of l: but so frustrating, when I want to be clear & to read. A curious throbbing this disease produces. But I've been on the whole vigorous and cheerful.[9]

In her novel *Mrs Dalloway* (1925), Woolf portrayed the menopause as an irrevocable sign of an 'end'.[10] Clarissa Dalloway embodies the contemporary attitudes and anxieties towards menopausal women of Woolf's generation: 'There was an emptiness about the heart of life; an attic room. Women must put off their rich apparel. At midday they must disrobe . . . narrower and narrower would her bed be', like the grave. Woolf allows Clarissa to confront these changing attitudes to her femininity, sexuality and identity and, finally, to 'have done with the triumphs of youth'.[11]

The female characters in the book (whose working title was *The Hours*, referring to 'the measuring out of human lives and seasons', a biological clock) cross all the seven ages of women: Clarissa and her friend Sally Seton are in their fifties; Clarissa's daughter, Elizabeth, is eighteen; Rezia Smith is in her twenties; Milly Brush and Doris Kilman are both in their forties; Millicent Bruton is sixty-two; Helena Parry in her eighties; and there is the lone elderly woman who lives opposite and whom Clarissa sees retiring to her solitary bed.

As Clarissa walked down Bond Street at the start of the day, Woolf has her musing on the wife of a friend, seeing doctors about a 'vague women's ailment':

> Of course, she thought, walking on, Milly is about my age –
> fifty, fifty-two. So it is probably *that*. Hugh's manner had said
> so, said it perfectly . . . How then could women sit in
> Parliament? How could they do things with men?

Tellingly, the original overt references to menstruation and menopause in this passage were eventually omitted from the final text. Even Clarissa's feeling for Sally, 'what men felt', is similarly opaquely rendered despite a growing openness about women's sexual feeling that had become apparent following the chaotic changes in political, social and economic spheres since the First World War.[12] Some women writers, finding their voices on the subject, were less 'sisterly' in their assessment of menopause and its impact on women and society. In American literature Lillian Smith's *Strange Fruit* (1944) portrays Alma, a doting white mother, as being unable to control herself or her children during her menopause, and in

Betty Smith's *A Tree Grows in Brooklyn* (1943) a woman regrets how few lovers she has had, as though her menopause will be the end of love and sex for her.[13] Change would be a long time coming.

Female medical writers toed the line too. Mary Chadwick, a state registered nurse, believed she was writing her book, *Woman's Periodicity* (London, 1933), on a subject that 'few people care to talk about'. Those who did talk about it were apt to ascribe to it 'every possible variety of unbalanced behaviour on the part of women, even when they are only nearing early middle-age'. Chadwick immediately added: 'occasionally they are right'. Women, she thought, 'begin to be anxious in secret about the future, and watch themselves apprehensively for peculiarities', as if everyone else checking them for such signs might not be enough. Even if they availed themselves of psychotherapy, the medical profession were fallible human beings, too, so consequently 'their thoughts and actions will be motivated by unconscious tendencies'. These negative attitudes would contribute to the general paucity of help and hostility towards menopausal women. Not surprisingly, many women had a 'grudge against life' and this, joined with the 'struggle to retain her youthful appearance' against a tide of 'caustic jokes or humourous articles in newspapers that are supposed to be of interest chiefly to men', made middle-age a very hard time for them.

Chadwick wasn't above giving them a hard time herself, but perhaps it had something to do with learned female self-deprecation on her part. 'We are often surprised,' she wrote, spitefully, 'when some amateur fortune-telling is in progress or Hallowe'en games are being played to see the most unlikely looking spinsters thrusting out their hands and asking coyly if they will be married.' This is especially harsh when we realize that these 'spinsters' were the young women who lost their men during the First World War. 'The approach of the menopause,' Chadwick continued, 'forces the realization that this hope is best abandoned.' How bleak and cruel. These women had lost the chance to love, marry, and perhaps have children and were considered to have lost their beauty and usefulness. They had become completely invalid objects of ridicule in the eyes of society. Even the influential Dame Mary Scharlieb MD had written how 'extremely pathetic' it is 'to find women well on to fifty years of age who are apparently as keen on sexual enjoyment as a bride might be'.

Even if she had been lucky enough to have had a child, a menopausal woman would be 'envious of her daughter's youth'. She could not win. Her envy would result in her resentment of 'the father and daughters going out together. They will plan pleasant projects', and her 'feeling of not being wanted or being shunned is typical of the climacteric woman. She will become very pathetic about it.' The early-twentieth-century menopausal woman in a nutshell: petty, critical, difficult, envious, bitter, resentful and obsessional – this, from a member of her own sex who had thoroughly imbibed the destructive assumptions that have been peddled for centuries. Chadwick even acknowledged the history, saying that the women's 'delusions remind us once again of the old-time witches . . . delusions of supreme importance and power'. 'Yet,' she wrote, unaware to the last, 'everyone at the time believed implicitly that what they thought was true, exactly like the women with their delusions of persecution alive today whose symptoms we have described.' She sees no parallel between her own ideas and those she marvels at; no wonder middle-aged women felt persecuted.

They had every reason to feel so, and every reason to greet Marie Stopes's book *Change of Life in Men and Women* with some relief. Stopes laid the blame for fear and loathing with medical practitioners who adversely stressed the natural changes, or apparent crises, in a woman's life in their popular works and were thus responsible for creating many of the very troubles they should have controlled. They had artificially created the crises by writing about women's 'disabilities' at this time and had emphasized 'a revolting, frightening, misleading and injurious state with a succession of the most lurid pictures of all the inevitable miseries which women were to anticipate'.[14] A ward sister at one of the 'world's most famous hospitals' told Stopes that nearly every case of menopausal difficulty she saw admitted to the hospital was induced by the ghastly things women had read and been told about what was going to happen. She felt that had they not 'met with such incitements to illness' they would probably have passed through the change with little or no difficulty. It was all falsity and hoodoo, yet gloomy anticipations of the menopause clouded the lives of many women, not only at the time of menopause itself but in anticipation, long before it arrived. Their health and happiness were overshadowed, generating fear which was in itself the very cause of the majority of the difficulties women experienced at this time. Stopes accused doctors, and gynaecologists in particular, of being incapable of imagining a healthy woman; they were all either fat and ugly or thin and dried-up and there was no mention of the 'happy mean, the ripening of the healthy, happy woman'.[15]

Doctors continued to regard hot flushes as a serious problem, even though they were the most common symptom a woman might complain of, and despite the fact that very little scientific work had been done on them. Stopes singled out Dr Hannan's work on *The Flushings of the Menopause*, wherein they were described as a somewhat neglected field. She declared herself astonished that women had had to wait until 1927 for an investigation of one of their most common experiences and even then only four patients were available for the medical research undertaken. Astonishing, too, that bloodletting, laughed out of existence a generation previously, was again returning to medical favour to deal with 'flushings'. The results of a survey by the Medical Women's Federation into menopausal symptoms published in the *Lancet* in January 1933 suggested that only 62 per cent of women actually experienced hot flushes. In the 1940s a 'maiden lady' aged nearly sixty said she felt they were an 'abomination of desolation', a married woman described the feeling of an impending flush as even worse than 'when you hear the cut out of a doodle-bomb', and yet another thought herself lucky to have her hot flushes at night as they kept her really warm in bed through the harsh winter of 1947.[16] To the women that did have them, hot flushes seemed to vary in intensity and timing and, not least, meaning. One anonymous female doctor thought that if it were possible for women to approach this phase of life without expecting any ill experiences then there would be little doubt that the average woman's discomforts would either be unnoticed or even considerably reduced.[17]

The Medical Women's Federation survey revealed that 15.8 per cent of menopausal women had no symptoms at all and 90 per cent had 'no interruption of work or routine due to any "symptoms"'. For the common complaint of sleeplessness Stopes recommended a good orgasm, the 'best soporific in the world', though women could avail themselves of sedatives if necessary, as long as they didn't indulge in morphia.

A morphia habit could bring on a premature menopause with all the 'discomforts of flushes and sweatings', according to Dr Arthur E. Giles, in his book *Sterility in Women* (London, 1919). This sounds more like withdrawal than a hot flush, but any confusion is hardly surprising as little was really understood about either addiction or menopause, and a symptom was a symptom, after all. For those who did suffer discomforts Stopes recommended a range of remedies, including: gland extracts, douching, bathing, electricity, calcium, iron, phosphates, sedatives, sulphur and 'rectal cleansing' as people were sometimes amazingly careless about their bowels: 'It should be realised that no one can be in perfect health who carries about a loaded rectum.' Dr Napier had suggested the use of electricity in the form of an inter-uterine electrode in 1897, and in 1903 a distinguished specialist is quoted as saying, sadly, that medical electricity occupied a humbler position in applied therapeutics than it deserved. But there were so many quacks and charlatans busy deceiving the public with their promises of a miracle cure with one electrical device or another that the medical profession was 'disposed to look askance at all such claims'. Stopes recommended her own device, on sale at her clinic at 108 Whitfield Street, London, W1, price five guineas, which conveniently plugged into any ordinary light fitting – where electricity had been installed. She did warn her readers, though, not to run off with the idea that any 'little "high-frequency" apparatus they may be offered in any shop will work all kinds of cures'. Personally, she would have liked to have seen such an apparatus in every intelligent person's home but thought the medical profession would, on the whole, object to 'unfettered access to self-help like this'.[18] It was suggested that electricity be combined with massage, diet and a sensible regimen to be truly beneficial. Still, in turn-of-the-century America electrotherapeutic equipment worth more than a million dollars was manufactured in over sixty establishments, mostly in New York and Illinois. At the time, the total value of electrical household goods was only about a fifth of this figure, and by 1914 sales were estimated to be about $2.6 million, so the controversy over efficacy wasn't putting the consumers off their buzz. Professional-looking equipment was advisable for physicians lest they lay themselves open to accusations of vulgarity by using the many consumer models that were available for home use. A good model of vibrator, not an obviously questionable massage machine, could be had for up to $75 in 1912 and the Chattanooga Vibrator, at the top end of the market, was selling at $200. The manufacturer suggested that, 'where the patient is a woman and the nervousness is caused by either the ovaries or uterus, particular attention should be given to the lower part of the spine and also to the affected organs themselves'. Dr Franklin Gottschalk thought the vibrator particularly useful for treating the menopause and recommended slow massages of 'fifty to one hundred periods per minute, giving muscles time to rest between each alternate contraction', and 'for sedation . . . a rapid vibration . . . seven to nine thousand periods per minute'.[19] One imagines he had a large and popular practice.

The most important, the most useful and, 'strange though it be, the most revolutionary advice' Stopes could give women was not to worry, to be the mistress of their emotions and to carry on exactly as though nothing special were happening. This was revolutionary. Almost everyone who published advice on this subject emphasized the 'need for all sorts of restrictions that the woman must impose upon

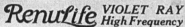
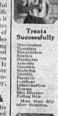

'Sugar-Coated Electricity' sent a 'warm, fresh blood surge' to any part of your body you fancied stimulating back to the 'vigor of youth'.

herself in her diet, her general habit and her pleasures'. Some of the punitive behaviours imposed by the pundits on menopausal women were 'monstrous'. She reiterated her message in bold:

Do not anticipate any trouble at all at this time.[20]

In fact, Stopes was of the opinion that things really began to look up after the menopause because so many women had written to her about an increase in their sexual feelings. One letter began:

> I am a widow with a grown up family, and since losing my husband a few years ago I so often have an active sexual feeling, and I wonder at my age (66), if it should be encouraged or repressed, or . . . if you could prescribe anything to give me just a little satisfaction at such times . . . I have always thoroughly enjoyed *conjugal* rights, but I should be glad to know if it is usual at my time of life to have such strong desires.

Another woman, a Mrs. D., aged fifty-one, had come to beg Stopes to tell her

> what she could do to renew the full married relations with her husband. She confessed that the fault was entirely hers. Two years previously her change of life had set in, and she thought she would never want anything more personally from married life. For a few months she was nervous and upset, and this confirmed the talk she had heard that 'everything was over' then. But soon she settled into a very easy and healthy time; to her surprise she felt far stronger and more vital than she had when the regular depletion of her

strength each month had continued. She now longed for
her husband's embraces, but remembered how she had
scolded him, and how emphatically she had assured him
that she would never want him as a husband in the physical
sense again. Now she was passionately longing to restore the
old happiness but was too shy to tell him so. Moreover he
had been brought up in a Christian home where he had been
taught that all sex life must cease when the wife's 'change'
came.[21]

The talk, suggestion, advice and rumour that sex ceases, or
should cease, at menopause was nothing more than a cultural sanction on desire, a fallacious and cruel device. One of
the earliest sex studies in the United States, begun in the 1890s
but not published until 1974 after its discovery in the Stanford
University archives, found that many of the post-menopausal
women questioned said they still enjoyed and wanted sex.
Clelia Mosher (1863–1940) began her research as a graduate
student at Wisconsin University with a questionnaire and lecture on marital relations given to the 'Mothers Club', a group
of faculty wives. Nearly fifty women completed the survey
and compellingly intimate material came from questions on
the 'true purpose of intercourse'. Thirty-three of the women
were born before 1870, thirteen of these before the Civil War
(1861–5), and many of the post-menopausal women in the
group told her that they still enjoyed and desired intercourse.[22] Stopes knew that denying this enjoyment and desire
caused great distress to many people and believed that the
nonsense about the menopause drove men to prostitution.
She considered it positively abominable and monstrous, a
moral madness which had arisen from the 'unwholesome-
ness of warped theological minds' and seduced educated and

otherwise sensible people to succumb to a stupid and ignorant piece of remorseless tyranny, a 'barbaric silliness masquerading as "religious virtue"'. Theological misconceptions had, she raged, dominated the medical mind to the detriment of women and men.

The Bishop of Southwark, for example, giving evidence to the Birth Rate Commission in 1915, stated that he had never been able to modify the view that the only thing that 'justifies ultimately the intercourse between the man and the woman is the purpose and desire to have children'. When he was asked if sex must cease after the possibility of the birth of children, he answered, 'I should say so.' If not, he loftily pronounced, the door would be wide open to a 'lowering of the whole idea of the union' and to the whole idea of the intercourse itself. Stopes thought that his insistence on the word 'lowering' was very revealing, and it is hard to disagree with her. This 'revolting' attitude also appeared in *The Conjugal Relationships* (New York, 1914), written by a Professor of Midwifery who argued that when the faculty of procreation was extinguished in women they were very soon degraded to the level of a being who has no further duty to perform in the world. And these pronouncements were being made in an age of high infant and maternal mortality and lack of contraception. It is difficult to see any humanity in this conflation of morality with physiology.

Dr Kisch, in *The Sexual Life of Women* (1910), was uncompromising in his stance on sex and the older woman: 'Among the stimulating influences which during the sexual epoch of the menopause are as far as possible to be avoided we must unhesitatingly include the practice of coitus.' And yet, he marvelled, it was 'precisely in women of the climacteric age [that] there often exists a strong desire'. This denial on the part of self-appointed physicians of women bred, according to Stopes, neuroses and psychological difficulties. Dr Kisch was, she thought, malign in his dismissal of a woman's sexual esteem. Malign and bound to the past, for he echoed Tilt in his role of physician-philosopher when he advised his peers to forbid any marriage between a woman 'in whom the menopause is drawing near' with a man who is 'still fully virile'. Disaster would surely follow as her 'sexual death is taking place'. Just as though, Stopes heatedly argued, woman is *only* a mother and her 'functions as mate, lover, and feminine individual with countless sex reactions came to an abrupt end!'[23]

In France, Professor Lacassagne, in the Parisian physician de Mussy's work *L'erotisme de la menopause*, discussed the 'trouble' of sexual arousal at the menopause, something 'which very probably is more common than the silence of gynaecologists would authorise us to suppose'. Again, the silence of the gynaecologists could have arisen from their ignorance as the aroused women, silenced by social mores, would not be rushing to consult their doctors. But, in America, Dr Emil Novak was saying in *Menstruation and its Disorders* (1931) that the menopause was just the end of the reproductive stage of a woman's life; not, 'as so many other doctors have it', the end of her sexual life.

Stella Browne believed that 'direct testimony from *various types* of women' was needed in order to understand the 'repressed sex-impulse [which] often breaks out irresistibly at the change of life, sometimes undermining sanity and control, through the remaining years. The happy memories and influences of a complete and active life, will always be a great safeguard through the critical years to a wise, healthy, kindly old age.' A Dr Drysdale, writing in the *Malthusian* in May 1915, suggested that 'the period of effective sexual life may be much extended by rational hygienic habits', and shortly afterwards Dr Mary Scharlieb, in the *British Medical Journal*, maintained that, anyway, the menopause was now occurring, on average, four or five years later than it had two generations ago. Browne's own conclusions were based 'on life, not books'. She attacked 'Pauline superstition', the double standard and conventional views and assumptions about women's sexuality as a denial of 'any strong, spontaneous, discriminating . . . sex impulse' in women, so that their sex life was 'merely a *response* to their husbands'. The idea that women were 'the private sex property of one man or the public sex property of all and sundry' amounted, she believed, to 'sadistic fetishism'.[24]

All depended on the individual woman, wrote Stopes, and not on a false social attitude that had created the pretence that a '"nice" married woman has herself no sex-hunger'.[25] It was the very height of wickedness, foolishness and cruelty to suggest that sexual desire in post-menopausal women was an indication of disease. Women must be 'freed from the piggery of nastiness created by the false idea that the end of physical love is enforced by the menopause . . . it is wasteful folly to throw people on the scrap heap of misery when they are in reality ripe for the enjoyment of life on a new basis'. She believed that the 'pomposities and patronising piffle' of some male physicians about menopausal women meant that they, and some priests, would have a great deal to answer for on the day of judgement. In 1922 Dr Walter Robie, an American sexologist, blamed most of the neuroses allegedly attending menopause on ignorance and false tradition; and Freud himself had noted that there was often a quite natural and healthy increase in 'sex feeling' in women at and after menopause. Stopes did acknowledge, too, that some women went off sex and their libido became dormant – a state she thought comparable with the temporary climacteric-impotence of many men. Some women, who had been, or even still were legally, wives, might be lonely and physically unsatisfied in their marriages and occasionally filled the void, as she put it, with a lesbian relationship. She supposed that this might take various forms and could actually be more popular than was generally recognized.

Any form of supposed deviant behaviour, so recently regarded as a moral insanity, contributed to many women's fears of 'losing mental control, even of becoming actually "insane" at the menopause'. This widespread fear of climacteric insanity was 'not based on true facts but . . . [on] widely credited gossip, and the malicious absurdities put into circulation by the nasty-minded'.[26] The figures of the lunacy commission in 1912 show that 8.2 per cent of all female asylum patients in England and Wales were committed with menopause as either a cause or an associated factor of their distress. Were the remaining 91.8 per cent there for similarly spurious reasons? In his book *The Woman Asks the Doctor* (London, 1936), Novak had argued that 'there is no scientific basis for the fear rather widely prevalent among intelligent women that the menopause is a common cause of insanity in women,' and 'the intelligent physician can render the mentally perturbed woman an inestimable service by rooting such beliefs from the back of her mind, where they have perhaps taken firm hold'. Radically, he exhorted doctors to be sympathetic and not 'ridicule' such anxieties, for a 'large proportion of women go through the menopause with scarcely a ripple', others may need a 'simple nerve sedative of some sort', and a minority 'the administration of certain "glandular" ovarian substances'.

Sympathy may have been too subjective a quality for many doctors, however. A decade after Novak's plea the psychologist Helene Deutsch, in her early sixties when she published a two-volume study, *The Psychology of Women*, in 1944–5, wrote of her own sex that, 'with the cessation of this function [menstruation] she ends her service to the species'. The 'organic decline' of menopause precipitated, she argued, a horrendously difficult period of psychologic adjustment.[27] Insomnia, anxiety states, excitability and depressions could all be provoked and determined by the deranged functioning of the endocrine system and woman's personality. Women struggle to preserve their femininity as 'all the forces of the ego are mobilized to achieve a better adjustment to reality, the old values crumble, and a drive to experience something new, exciting, makes itself felt'. Some experienced a strong urge to become pregnant, some turned to occupations 'outside their homes', some revived 'long-buried' interests given up when they married. It might seem like a transformation, a period of adjustment to a new phase of life, but the message was most definitely mixed. The menopausal woman was in the grip of a 'narcissistic mortification' as her 'beauty-creating activity' declined, a 'gradual loss of femininity' overwhelmed her, she felt the 'threatened devaluation' of her genitals and perceived the 'first signs of old age'. All of this disastrous-sounding process served, unfortunately, to heighten her interest in herself. About time, some of us might think.

Any benefit a woman might have derived from her menopause was squashed beneath the weight of Deutsch's language and professional certainty: menopause was nothing less than a 'partial death'. Even if Deutsch allowed for 'higher brain centres and a complicated emotional life that was not restricted to motherhood' any 'proof that she is biologically alive' came from menstruation, and without that she experienced increased aggression and depressive moods due to the 'loss that for a woman is equivalent to castration'. The 'whole female genital apparatus' was reduced to 'inactive and superfluous structures', all 'beauty vanishes, and usually the warm, vital flow of feminine emotional life as well'.

Reduced, too, to a 'second puberty', a 'preclimacterical thrust' brings increased sexual excitement and readiness and 'respectable' people could be 'very much surprised' by a menopausal woman's behaviour in all its tragic-comic oddities. Her intensified sexual feeling 'usually does not go farther than self-gratification' as women 'revive the clitoris masturbation they long ago gave up' (apparently) and this was 'especially true of old maids without any direct genital experience', those, presumably, who had no man to show them how it should be done properly. Calling on Freud and echoing the ancient notion of the male body as norm, Deutsch argued that puberty and menopause were analogous 'because in both cases masculinity is given up in the attempt to become a woman' and this 'usually fails in the climacterium'. What she termed 'feminine-loving women' she deemed to have a milder menopause than 'masculine-aggressive ones', and those 'who have lived in a harmonious, happy, sexually gratifying marriage, enjoy the late storms in its calm haven'. Unlike 'ridiculous old women [they] enjoy their erotic gifts to the end'.

For the unlucky 'masculine-aggressive' woman it was a dangerous age and even if she had 'previously avoided violent experiences, she is suddenly seized by an urge to make her life richer, more active'. Horror – she might start a diary, get into 'abstract ideas' and might even leave home. Although the 'chances' of older women improved because men sensed

that they would make 'lesser demands upon their masculinity', their use of cosmetics and fashion made them behave like
girls and they fell prey to a 'narcissistic self-delusion' where
'her painted face appears youthful to her in the mirror'. She
would forget all her experience and 'at the age of 50 she is
absolutely unready to renounce anything'. All this startlingly
spiteful judgmental language, dressed up as medical fact,
drew on centuries of social censure and disapproval, almost
unmitigated by the actual experiences of women in the
Western world in the mid-1940s. The Freudian balm of 'love
for one's own person [as] perhaps the secret of beauty', a 'psychic cosmetic' that cannot be replaced by 'rouge, massages,
and youthful dress', is perhaps a tricky thing to pull off when
you are a pointless castrate suffering partial death.

Deutsch suggested, ironically, that good judgement
deserted the women she was writing about. She accused them
of surrounding themselves with inferior men in order to be
admired, becoming boastful, becoming interested in 'disrep-
utable' women, believing that their marriage was a 'degrading
mistake', and digging up old letters from former lovers, they
were hysterically 'driven to act out their fantasies'. It's difficult
to decide if this is worse than the alternative which, she said,
involved aestheticism, philanthropy, religion, self-sacrifice
and the life of a 'pious bigot'. Then there would be a retreat
into 'splendid isolation' to protect herself from her frustrations and, at worst, her friendships might become 'troubled',
or she might experience a 'homosexual panic'. The menopause, according to Deutsch, had a psychogenic 'twilight state
[that] brings to light what lies at the bottom of the soul',
which appeared to render a woman for ever child-like and
prey to her biological self.

For women to think otherwise was still considered by some

as misguided into the 1960s. Dr Elizabeth Parker had advised graceful acceptance, for a 'rebellious woman is certain to be an unhappy woman . . . doomed to failure, since she cannot stay the natural cycle of life' and this rebellion is rooted in her 'immaturity and ignorance'. Parker's work *The Seven Ages of Women* was written specifically for women so, following her beliefs, she made sure the 'scientific technicalities and language have been eliminated as far as possible', tainting her otherwise straightforward information and occasional enlightening idea with the deadening effect of established and patronizing cultural mores. She suggested it was 'formidable', for example, to attempt to 'explain' femininity and its 'mysteries'; indeed, the subtitle of *The Seven Ages of Women* shouts 'WOMAN – THE ETERNAL MYSTERY!' as Parker swallows and regurgitates stale male dogma. Women, she reasoned, have

> never been the dominant sex in government or commerce, war or exploration, science, or even the arts . . . we might well ask why this is so. She has intelligence, imagination, and determination . . . the one quality for success in these areas of human endeavour that she seems to have lacked is interest. Perhaps, therefore, she occupies her position from choice. To her, fulfilment was not to be measured in terms of success and the furtherance of what we are pleased to call progress and civilisation but in the intangibles of human relationships, and she found it good to be a woman. Her eagerness, her interest has always been directed towards this – the perfection of her femininity.[28]

Beginning from a position of culturally defined femininity, Parker dressed up the hoary old argument of nature, again, for modern consumption.

Serenity, moderation, acceptance of a diminished role and a disinterest in sex are menopausal 'virtues' that have seeped into our present but began to be questioned openly by women during the twentieth century. In 1948 a female gynaecologist who felt the need to write under the pseudonym 'Medica' published *Change of Life: Facts and Fallacies of Middle Age* and dedicated it (with some condescension) 'To a little housemaid who once contemplated suicide because she had been told that her hot flushes were a sign of a very guilty conscience.' 'Medica' knew that 'ignorance and superstition die hard; and they retain their grip relentlessly on . . . the change of life'.[29] That same year Dr Josephine Barnes gave a series of talks on radio about the health of older women. Dame Josephine (1912–99) was an obstetrician and gynaecologist, the first FRCOG to give birth and the first woman president of the British Medical Association. She was immensely influential and worked at the women-only Elizabeth Garrett Anderson Hospital until she retired in 1977, later helping to save it from closure. In her radio broadcasts she discussed blood loss, ovaries, hormonal changes during the menopause and uterine cancers and sent the head of the Home Service into a tail-spin: 'The inclusion of such a talk represents a lowering of broadcasting standards. It is acutely embarrassing to hear about hot flushes, diseases of the ovary and the possibility of womb removal transmitted . . . at two o'clock in the afternoon.'[30] Janet Quigley, who became editor of *Woman's Hour* in 1950, sent a memo to the controller of talks on 16 March 1956 outlining her editorial philosophy: to bring 'hush-hush' topics into the open, 'so that the less-educated amongst our listeners may get used to the idea that no subject which concerns them as citizens need be taboo'. She had introduced items on child guidance, loneliness, divorce, marital difficulties (which the *Daily Mirror* thought was the 'frankest ever talk' when the 'intimate side of wedlock was mentioned') and the menopause. This last subject, however, could not be broadcast during the school holidays.

Embarrassment, censure and distaste were still apparent in the 1970s when Donald Carr published *The Sexes*. It was all 'rather revolting', he thought, this 'ovary degeneration' and these 'pseudo-testicles'. The foul 'sex reversal' he was describing happened to hens but it was nonetheless an 'ugly metamorphosis . . . not unknown among mammals, including men' – or women, we must presume he meant. The process in birds was, he said, 'sufficiently common that in the Middle Ages crowing hens were considered bewitched and immediately had their necks wrung, and their bodies burned and the ashes scattered over water', a behaviour also not unknown amongst men. Menopause was just a revolting metamorphosis, an intrinsically 'bad' change. Carr seems to have been caught in something of a bind where menopause was concerned, appalled by the fact of it and furious with the meaning of it in religious and personal terms:

The existence in human females simultaneously of menopause and of sexuality continuing *after* menopause introduces a seemingly insoluble dilemma for some of the more stubborn policy makers of the Catholic Church. The arguments against artificial contraception are based on the so-called 'natural law', i.e., that the act of sex was designed to create babies and that any hampering of this purpose is therefore a crime against the 'natural law' . . . harsh objection is obviously applicable to the intercourse of a woman beyond the menopause . . . In such cases the man is theologically doing the same thing as going through the motions of

copulating with another man, an animal of another species
or even with a pillow. It is obvious that in refusing to look
upon intercourse as an act of love the Church has, in effect,
renounced the idea of love between the sexes and reduced
intercourse to a purely biological transaction which we share
with all bisexual animals. In other words, the Church, orig-
inally founded upon the idea of the unique spirituality of
man, has now painted itself and its faithful flocks into a
corner with the monkeys and the squirrels.[31]

Fear, disgust and confusion were still lurking just below the
surface of even the most rational-seeming medical and scientific texts, influenced as they must be by the social,
religious, economic and political status quo, as well as the
accumulated ideology stretching from the ancient idea of
the male as the norm and the female as a pathological deviation from it.

Robert Wilson's message of 'unpalatable truth', the decay
and 'defeminization' of menopause and the grey-veiled existence of 'harmless docile creatures missing most of life's
values' had still managed to sway some in the early feminist
movement with the promise of being 'fully sexed', or at least
fully alive, on HRT. But the disease model of menopause and
hormonal 'cure' was problematical: should women shun
medicalization or should they demand even more medical
attention for their particular needs; was this medical innovation a help or a hindrance to women's liberation; should
women control their own bodies or seize apparently greater
control with hormones? Feminists were caught between
accusing the medical system of treating women as inherently sick and accusing them of not appreciating how sick
women might be.[32]

Surprisingly, there is little feminist research on when menopause occurs, how long it lasts, and how medical definitions of menopause affect the individual woman. Feminist scholars working in this field have concentrated mostly on social contexts and not directly challenged the biomedical definitions and doctors' diagnoses, and, where they have, their audience has been limited. Not that biological factors in menopause should be denied, rather there shouldn't be an exclusive focus on the psychological and sociocultural factors. Part of menopause does, of course, rest on established age- and time-based definitions and these affect how women feel about it and how medicine responds to them.[33] And feminists didn't always agree between themselves – some greeting HRT as a gift for ageing women and others seeing it as defining them as diseased and requiring treatment. Attitudes changed when, in 1975, the studies linking HRT and endometrial cancer were published, but this didn't mean complete consensus. It did, though, bring in a wider agenda for women's health, particularly emphasizing the need for women to retain control of their bodies and participate fully in the decision-making efforts regarding their health.

Menopause came in from the periphery. Belle Canon, the American research scientist and writer, thought the HRT controversy gave 'the first and only stimulus to public and medical discussion of menopause' and that women would no longer have to 'weather the storm'[34] (assuming there was a real storm to be weathered). Wendy Cooper, a British journalist, saw HRT as allowing women to control the biology that had controlled them for so long. She used the words of Dr Francis Rhoades as 'splendid ammunition': 'The physician should not let inherent male resentment of female longevity and biological superiority deter him from his medical responsibility. Because men do not experience the dramatic and often devastating changes represented by the menopause, they have come to regard it as normal for women to suffer [its] consequences.'[35] Women would now be free to compete with men on equal terms. Even though many thought that the 'problems' of the menopause were 'responses to the society's evaluation of the older woman's status' they still embraced 'oestrogen deficiency' as a valid explanation. The anthropologist Paula Weideger, in her book *Menstruation and Menopause: The Physiology and Psychology, the Myth and the Reality* (1976), wrote that women just had to 'live with the results of nature's error' and should accept the help of medical technology. She did note, though, that 'any woman who now chooses ERT, is a guinea pig and a gambler'.[36]

Doctors, obstetricians and gynaecologists (women doctors could also hold misogynistic views) discussed the changing attitudes of their patients: 'What is behind these demands that threaten the staid orderliness of the doctors' office . . . What do these women want?' asked the *American Medical News* in 1974 in an article entitled 'And Now, the "Liberated" Woman Patient'. Feminists were arguing that the answer to menopausal difficulties was a change in women's attitudes to their ageing bodies and in women's role in society. Menopause was a natural phenomenon, not a disease, and women were urged to break out of their socially sanctioned roles. Rosetta Reitz's book *Menopause: A Positive Approach* (1977) laid out the new feminist positions. 'I accept,' she wrote, 'that I'm a healthy woman whose body is changing. No matter how many articles and books I read that tell me I'm suffering from a "deficiency disease", I say I don't believe it. I have never felt more in control of my life than I do now and I feel neither deficient nor diseased.' Feminism was giving women the freedom to question their experience at the hands of the medical profession.[37]

In the early 1980s McKinlay and McKinlay reported on a survey of over 8000 random women aged 45–55 saying that the 'vast majority' of middle-aged women did not express regret at reaching the menopause, did not report more symptoms or poorer health, and did not increase their use of health services. Younger, peri-menopausal women were 'more concerned about experiencing menopause than were women who were actually menopausal or post-menopausal'.[38] If HRT was designed in part, wittingly or not, to nullify women with artificial menses, a psychosomatic passivity and a yoke of fake youth, the new psychosexual model of the menopause that emerged in the 1980s would help to turn the tables and incorporate the feminist agenda. The new clinical model would provide a 'multidisciplinary team approach', the patient's symptoms and complaints would be clearly specified and, further, it would be necessary to go beyond them and discover her personal perceptions and meanings of menopause, including a history of any 'previous adversity, particularly during other critical phases of her life'. Finally, all this 'must be evaluated in the context of her total socio-cultural milieu . . . it is perhaps the responsibility of the clinician to construct the truly integrative model in the person of the individual woman'.[39] It's not difficult to see Fothergill's eighteenth-century approach to the menopause in this, borne out by the new cynical promotion of the use of hormones as symptom management and as a prophylactic against old age.

9

FEAR OR FREEDOM

Many women have told me that the much dreaded menopause, being over, they were delighted to find that it had not been nearly so bad as they had expected. *Fear* of the event had been universally worse than the facts of the change when once it came upon them. Fear not only clouds natural happiness in the present in anticipation of a dreaded future, it has the power to create the very thing its victim dreads.

Marie Stopes, *Change of Life in Men and Women*

The menopause has been thoroughly medicalized in Western culture and this process has determined the way we now think of, respond to, and feel about it. We have to look to its medical history to understand why this natural phenomenon has become sodden with a cultural negativity which is ill-founded and spurious. My initial embarrassment at researching this book turned to anger as I realized the shame, suspicion and mockery that has attended women in mid-life – misery which began with the earliest medical attitudes to the female body. The principles of Greek and Roman medicine were still being followed in the West in the eighteenth century. Add religious ideals to these preconceptions of the 'viler sex' as deformed males, interesting only as breeders, and it's clear why such fear and distaste surrounds the older and menopausal woman. With or without science or orthodox medicine, society will express attitudes to the female body through myths, superstitions and folklore and some of medicine's answers may seem just as fantastic as the irrational notions it has sought to overturn. Powerful medico-cultural trends have dictated women's experience of the menopause and how much they, in turn, have surrendered to, resisted, or influenced them. There are many tensions between sex, science and sensibility, and many passionate medics and writers to argue over them.

The story of the menopause has covered difference, divinity, wandering wombs, cunning women, lustiness, suspicion, sex, surgery, manliness, madness, power, irrationality, seclusion, collusion and the whole ageing question with its attendant public and private anxieties. The combination of sex, power and knowledge is its benefit, yet claims of pathology, deviation and invisibility are its cultural parameters. Yet the menopause has never been an uncommon experience. Historically, if you made it past puberty and childbirth, you stood a very good chance of reaching old age. More and more women now spend longer in the post-menopausal period than ever before, at least in the West, yet they seem to be more and more fearful. This is the tragedy and this is why perceptions of the menopause have to be revised. It isn't an end, it is just another event in ordinary female life.

The history of the menopause has run from, at best, ignoring it, to the earliest proponents of managing symptoms, to the beginnings of medicalization and the advent of science, to the controversies of hormone drug therapies. Recently the pendulum has swung back to management, as illustrated by the publication of *Managing the Menopause without Oestrogen*, which received a Highly Commended award in the Obstetrics and Gynaecology category in the 2005 BMA Book Awards. It was published by the British Menopause Society, a registered charity that is dedicated to 'meeting the challenge of the menopause'. The menopause, we note, is still considered a 'challenge' – which might be acceptable if the challenge being faced was the combined power of disease, ageism, sexism and the many other medico-cultural assumptions, rather than the phenomenon itself.

The medical construction of the menopause and the treatments that were subsequently devised and prescribed were less a conspiracy than part of the unpredictable development of a scientific fact – the uncertainties, controversies and decision-making which sprang from the overall 'rise of science' from the eighteenth century onwards. Mary Wollstonecraft (1759–97), in her introduction to *A Vindication on the Rights of Women*, remarked on a 'lively writer, I cannot recollect his name', who asked 'what business women turned of forty have to do in the world'. It was this sort of prevailing ideology which informed the approach of the physicians of the day as they treated older women.

The philosopher Karl Popper (1902–94) wrote that science is a biological phenomenon which has arisen out of pre-scientific knowledge; it is a remarkable continuation of commonsense knowledge. Science, he wrote, 'starts from *problems*, from *amazement* about something that might be quite ordinary in itself [original emphasis]'.[1] The menopause was perceived as a problem when women presented to their physicians or were told that it was one, but it was hardly amazing to the women themselves.

As the anthropologist Mary Douglas has said, we cannot possibly interpret our beliefs and assumptions unless 'we are prepared to see in the body a symbol of society, and to see the powers and dangers credited to social structures reproduced in small on the human body'. Taboo, she says, is a device for fencing and protecting distinctive categories of life and the world about us.[2] Anthropological cross-cultural studies of the menopause reveal a great variety of perceptions, meanings and taboos depending on cultural practices, myths and symbols. In some cultures, including India, Mexico, Greece and China, where women gain status as they age, the menopause is not associated with disease or dysfunction.[3] Modern Jewish Orthodox practice has recently begun to address the great silence surrounding the menopause by creating new rituals, and this change is driven by women themselves.[4] Buddhism, which places emphasis on the impermanence of life, teaches women to accept easily the menopause and all the changes that occur throughout their lives. But there is growing evidence that the increased interest of doctors, in Thailand for example, is shifting traditional and popular perceptions of the menopause as a culturally valued, natural event; it has begun to be seen as a negative, biomedical problem.[5]

Until recently, orthodox medicine believed that HRT was 'an extremely safe' treatment for vasomotor symptoms, osteoporosis, peri-menopausal depression, loss of energy and libido, and a major preventative measure for heart disease, colon cancer and Alzheimer's. Pro-HRT doctors still peddle this view. The 'challenge', according to Professor John Studd, chairman of the British Menopause Society, is to find an oestrogen or oestrogen-like hormone which protects the skeleton, cardiovascular system, the brain and the breast, while producing 'enough positive symptomatic benefits that women are *happy to remain on the therapy for many years* [my italics]'. After the early cancer scares of the 1970s, heavy promotion by pharmaceutical companies of 'safer' combinations of oestrogen and progestin led to an increase in the use of HRT. In 1992 17 per cent of women over fifty years old were taking the drugs and this figure doubled to 33 per cent in 2001.

Then, in 2002, the Women's Health Initiative (WHI), a fifteen-year research study of over 161,000 post-menopausal women aged 50–79 being conducted in America, stopped its HRT trials three years early because of the overall health risks it uncovered: the risks of invasive breast cancer and cardiovascular disease were exceeding the benefits of the drug. Its findings were headline news. Major medical authorities changed their tack, saying HRT should be used only in cases of severe symptoms and only for very short periods. In panic, many women opted out and numbers of prescriptions written fell dramatically, by 43 per cent.[6] Nearly half of the 1.7 million women in Britain and the 22 million women in America who were taking HRT came off the treatment. The US Food and Drug Administration (FDA) introduced the highest level of warning on the boxes of the drugs, highlighting the increased risks for heart disease, heart attacks, strokes and breast cancer, and emphasizing that they are not approved for heart disease prevention and should be used only when the benefits clearly outweigh the risks. The WHI has its critics, who say that the research was flawed and that millions of women have come off HRT needlessly. Evaluating the risks and the benefits and defining the differences between a symptomatic and an asymptomatic woman, however, have never been straightforward tasks. Critics argue that the WHI findings related to women whose average age was sixty-three — ten years older than the average age for menopause — and had these women been given HRT in their fifties they could possibly have been afforded some protection against cardiovascular disease. Pharmaceutical companies, fearing major financial losses, increasingly emphasize in advertising and promotional material fears of ageing and, yes, death.

Other studies, reporting at the same time as the WHI, also found that HRT didn't have a beneficial effect on heart disease as claimed. In January 2006 a paper published in the *British Journal of Obstetrics and Gynaecology* (*BJOG*) reported that 'despite decades of evidence from observational studies, the use of hormone therapy for the prevention of cardiovascular disease among postmenopausal women is controversial.' The review of the latest available trial data revealed that hormone therapy does not significantly change their risk of coronary heart disease but that it does increase their risk of stroke.[7]

Alzheimer's and other dementias are another area of contention in the HRT debate. In 2008 BBC News reported that women have a higher risk of developing Alzheimer's than men and, according to London's Institute of Psychiatry, HRT might protect post-menopausal women against it. The theory is that oestrogen helps to prevent the build-up of damaging protein tangles in the brain which are thought to aggravate the disease, so when supplies of the hormone lessen women may become more vulnerable. The Alzheimer's Society was more circumspect, saying that 'using HRT as a treatment or preventative measure against Alzheimer's disease would mean giving drugs, which can have side-effects, to women without symptoms'. The Alzheimer's Research Trust found no conclusive evidence and advised women not to start HRT specifically to protect against dementia because of HRT's side-effects and the increased risk of stroke.

Another risk factor in taking the hormone replacements is breast cancer. The Million Women Study (MWS), set up to investigate the effects of specific types of HRT on breast cancer, is the largest of its kind in the world. Between 1996 and 2001, one in four women in the UK aged 50–64 years was recruited. Nearly 950,000 women took part. They provided information about their use of HRT and other personal details and were followed up for cancer incidence and death for an average of almost seven years. Around a third of the women were taking HRT and a further fifth had taken it in the past. The MWS found that use of HRT by these women over the past decade has resulted in an estimated 20,000 extra breast cancers and that the therapy is seen as the principal avoidable risk for this disease.[8] More than 44,000 women are diagnosed with breast cancer in Britain every year. The numbers have increased by more than 12 per cent over the past decade – and by more than 80 per cent since 1971. On present trends, the total could reach 58,000 annually by 2024, according to Cancer Research UK. HRT may also have caused the deaths of more than 1000 women in the UK from ovarian cancer since 1991 – one woman in 2500 will get ovarian cancer while a long-term user of HRT, and one in every 3300 will die from it. When the use of HRT declined it was thought that this did bring a lowering of breast cancer rates in the USA.

For fifty years HRT use has been increasing in our society yet even nearly thirty years ago worries about endometrial cancer led the National Institute of Aging to state that HRT 'is only effective in the treatment of hot flushes and vaginal atrophy, and if used at all, should be administered on a cyclical basis (three weeks of oestrogen, one week off) at the lowest dose for the shortest possible time'.[9] This advice remained constant among many authorities. Yet pharmaceutical companies pushed HRT and certain doctors have been loud advocates. Like other treatments over the ages, HRT has been pushed on women without full knowledge in response to misogynistic ideas about what women should be and want. Professor John Toy, Cancer Research UK's medical director, has said recently that women should think very carefully about whether to take HRT, and if they choose to take it they should do so for clear medical need and for the shortest possible time.[10]

Professor Mayur Lakhani, chairman of the Council of the Royal College of General Practitioners, speaking on the BBC in 2007, argued that there are no long-term benefits of taking HRT and that he would not prescribe it for longer than a year. All the risks, which appreciate by duration of treatment, needed to be taken into account as, in his opinion, it is clinically hard to justify keeping a woman on HRT for decades. Responding to this, Professor Studd argued that anything from five to fifteen years was a common length of time to take HRT and that many of his patients have been taking it for twenty years and don't want to stop. Mr Peter Bowen-Simpkins, consultant and spokesperson for the Royal College of Obstetricians and Gynaecologists, thought that five years is considered a reasonable time on HRT and blamed the media for giving the general public an attack of nerves over hormones by being cavalier in their use and explanation of statistics. Studd agreed, saying that the press had done women an injustice by frightening them off HRT.[11]

Interestingly, a report on British female general practitioners revealed that 50 per cent of those taking HRT are still on it twenty years after starting, so they obviously feel that the risks are worth taking and that using the drugs for decades is acceptable.[12] In an HRT debate on BBC Radio 4's *Woman's Hour* in 2007, Eileen Marshall, aged eighty, who took HRT for twenty-eight years, said she would still be taking it now if she could. Recounting how much she disliked what she said were menopausal symptoms – feeling depressed and lethargic – she visited her doctor, who first prescribed valium. When this drug didn't suit her she tried HRT. Asked whether she hadn't thought that her hot flushes and other symptoms would pass and whether she had been concerned by possible side-effects of taking the drugs, Eileen replied that it was a chance she had been willing to take. She had felt so low and depressed she would have done anything to get over that stage in her life. She recalled that on HRT she had felt much better, had more vitality, and had gone skiing, climbing, travelling – all this, perhaps pertinently, after she had been widowed. She stopped taking HRT only when her doctor told her that at her age it wasn't giving her any more benefit. However, in one study undertaken at a general practice in Britain, 80 per cent of women taking HRT for menopausal symptoms said they would have liked to have had more information about the menopause before it happened to them and only 5 per cent of them had actually requested the therapy.[13] It seems that the apparent control and convenience that HRT promises women is a delusion, and a costly one at that.

There are medical alternatives to HRT: calcium, for example, is recommended, based on studies which have shown that about 1.5G of elemental calcium is necessary to preserve bone health in post-menopausal women not taking HRT; and selective serotonin-reuptake inhibitors, which are said to be effective in treating hot flushes. And there are plenty of other alternative therapies for the menopause which have expanded as part of a popular backlash against orthodox medicine, in the tradition of self-treating women. The extent and nature of the business, which has its own vested interest in the menopause as a treatable disease of 'lack', is huge. Herbal remedies and other complementary medicines and therapies include black cohosh,[14] kava kava, dong quai, evening primrose, ginkgo biloba, gingseng, St John's wort, liquorice root and valerian, diet and vitamin supplements, acupressure, acupuncture, the Alexander technique, Ayurveda, osteopathy, hypnotherapy, reflexology, reiki, Tai Chi and homeopathy. Chinese medicine recognizes an increased incidence of menopause-related symptoms as being related to modern Western lifestyles but doesn't recommend HRT, believing it makes women feel better only in the short term and actually exacerbates the depletion of the body's resources.[15]

All these products and processes are sold to women to ease them over what they have been taught to think of as a traumatic, unpleasant and unfair event in their lives. It plays into the need to remain desirable, valid and potent. How much that need is a cynical marketing construct is open to argument. Surely health and independence are the most important and fundamental needs and from these follow desirability and validity. You could be forgiven for thinking that today the menopause boils down, as so many things seem to, to drugs and sex, to the presence or absence, quality or quantity of either. Historically, absurd assumptions that sex stops, or should stop, at the menopause have had serious implications for the treatment, health and well-being of post-menopausal women. Research by groups such as the Pennell

Initiative for Women's Health, a charity campaigning for the needs of women over the age of forty-five that has commissioned research into sexuality and the menopause, is trying to rectify the mistakes. The Pennell study of 2001 attempted to demystify what for many remains a taboo subject and to show that sex is important to many older women. According to the report a menopausal woman is more likely to eschew penetrative sex in favour of other more sensual or tactile experiences and her answers would skew any research project which followed the conventional idea of sex being solely concerned with penetration. Whilst it is true that the capacity to reproduce ends at the menopause, and that vaginal lubrication can decrease, they say that 'women's sexual arousal or orgasm capacity actually increases'. In 2006 an American study on 'Sexual Activity and Function in Middle-aged and Older Women' reported in *Obstetrics and Gynaecology* on the experiences of 'sexual activity, frequency, satisfaction and dysfunction' of a diverse group of just over 2000 women aged between forty and sixty-nine years of age. Their average age was 55.9 years and nearly three fourths of them were sexually active. According to Shere Hite's latest work, *The New Hite Report* (2000), older women are 'more likely to enjoy more multiple orgasms than younger women' and 'confusion between reproductive activity and sexual pleasure is playing havoc with our lives'. We need to stop repeating outdated assumptions about older women.

If some women experience a diminution of 'aggressive sexual desire', something which comes under definitions of female sexual dysfunction (FSD), they may or may not be content with this change. Science is a clumsy tool with which to describe subjective experience, and individual response can be, at the very least, marginalized. If women report a loss of libido they may find themselves being treated to maintain a higher level of libido through drugs despite an incompatibility with other aspects of their mid-life experience. Despite, too, the huge problems in validating data where they have been collected, and the difficulties in defining 'libido' and 'dysfunction', which are based mainly on 'genitally focused events in a linear sequence model', i.e. desire, arousal and orgasm (so narrow, so inadequate, so unlike the experience of many women for whom it runs: desire, arousal, second thoughts).

Historically the menopause has attracted the language of loss, decline and decay while spermatozoa have been rewarded with the language of vitality. Not much seems to have changed. Fertility expert Robert Winston, talking at the Cheltenham Science Festival in 2007, discussed the development of a pill which would extend the life of a woman's eggs using proteins to protect them, and delay her menopause: 'What we are seeing,' he said, 'is increasingly a society where women are . . . getting educated and careers . . . but their biology is working against them.' He told his audience that, in the time they had been listening to him, 'every woman of child-bearing age [here] will have lost two eggs', adding, 'by contrast, I will have made 150,000 new sperm'. He must have produced absolutely millions by now. Well done him.

The drive to retain youth, desirability and potency leads some women to submit eagerly to the surgeon's knife. Max Beerbohm's (1872–1956) vacuous remark in A Defence of Cosmetics that 'women are not so young as they are painted' could be rewritten now as 'not so young as they are sculpted'. In 2007 there were over 32,400 cosmetic surgery procedures performed in the UK, up by 12.2 per cent from 2006, according to the report of the British Association of Aesthetic Plastic Surgeons (BAAPS).[16] Facelifts had the largest increase among all procedures, up by 36 per cent (4468 procedures carried out), keeping their place as the fourth most popular choice. The majority of the work was carried out on women (91 per cent), who underwent 29,572 procedures. The top choice for women continues to be breast augmentation, with 6497 operations. Male surgery increased by 17.5 per cent, with 2881 surgical procedures (compared with 2452 in 2006). The male-grooming market added up to £685 million in 2004 and, according to Mintel, the market analysts, men will be spending £821 million in 2009. BAAPS reported that other anti-ageing procedures continued to show a steady rise in popularity for both men and women, increasing by 13 per cent and 11 per cent overall. According to Mr Douglas McGeorge, consultant plastic surgeon and president of BAAPS, the audit for 2007 clearly reflects Britain's 'continued acceptance of aesthetic surgery, particularly in the area of anti-ageing'. BAAPS also suggested, in a paper on the psychological aspects of aesthetic surgery, that over 50 per cent of Botox users 'expressed a lack of control over the natural ageing process', and over 50 per cent reported actually 'feeling' younger rather than just 'looking' younger.

The French novelist Colette founded a beauty parlour in Paris in the 1930s and spent four hours a day, five days a week there, believing that older women should not break the 'contract they signed with beauty'. 'Since I have cared for and made up my contemporaries,' she wrote, 'I have not yet met a fifty-year-old woman who was discouraged . . . The harder the times for women, the more the woman, proudly, insists on hiding that she suffers'.[17] Americans spend up to $15 billion a year on cosmetic surgery, double the gross domestic product of Malawi and over twice the American contribution to AIDS programmes in the past decade.[18] Annual spending on women's cosmetics in Britain has risen by 40 per cent in the past five years, to more than £1 billion. A survey commissioned by British cosmetics manufacturer Dove, which uses naked women over fifty to advertise its pro-age products, revealed that 89 per cent of older women believe that the media fails to portray their age group accurately and contributes to its denigration and invisibility. This 'need' to remain visible is reflected in increasing numbers of treatments and potions, which include the liver flush, colonic enemas, Botox and proprietary products such as StriVectin, for those 'stubborn surface imperfections'. This Klein-Becker product claims to be a 'deep wrinkle serum' targeting that 'dynamic interface [at the] dermal-epidermal junction', and at a cost of $153 for a 0.9 ounce bottle (approximately twenty-eight applications), it ain't cheap! The publicity proclaims: *'This year it's all about the hands!'*, as though your hands are a fashion accessory, so they won't have to look 'old, veiny and embarrassing'. All this frantic promotion, activity and anxiety-mongering is in pursuit of the eradication of ugliness, and our society sees older bodies as ugly. Our preoccupation with appearance seems to suggest that while we shun the prospect of getting old we are much more afraid of getting ugly.[19]

If we remove the established constraints of medicine and culture, the menopause is simply one more feature in a woman's linear life history, an inevitable and natural phenomenon that follows on from her beginning in the womb, her birth, puberty, adolescence and pregnancy. Viewed in this light, the menopause and post-menopause will cease to inspire anxiety. It is just one more change to negotiate, and nowhere near as astonishing or potentially problematic as pregnancy. If we come to change our negative perceptions of it then its cultural meaning will change too, and some of the ingrained prejudices against older women will fall away.

The historian Edward Shorter recently wrote about the historically unequal status of women resulting from victimization by their reproductive organs. It doesn't seem to have registered that reproductive organs do not victimize anyone; people and cultures do that. Here is a modern historian reinforcing the idea of women as biologically determined, inherently vulnerable victims, 'deeply debased and humiliated' by their bodies, which have forced them into an inevitable contract with 'patriarchy'. It is as if patriarchy, too, were biologically, naturally, determined. The impressive achievements of medical science and the less impressive achievements of some commentators continue to mirror older cultural and religious assumptions about women. But if menopausal 'normality' was largely defined by the attitudes and interpretations of male physicians, medicine was practised differently in the past. It will be practised differently in the future.[20]

So much depends on how you view your own menopause, and you must be able to see and analyse what society makes of it to reject the negativity that has stuck like the filthiest thick mud to this natural phenomenon. We can move on from the early-twentieth-century endocrine perverts and derailed menopausics, leaving the prejudices behind. Unless a woman is struggling badly with the consequences of the menopause so that her quality of life is really diminished, the future of the menopause lies in self-management as it did in the past, not in a doctor-delivered cure. Talk to women who are going through or have been through it. Ask them what they think and know about it. Take this as your guide. The point, surely, is the freedom, as de Beauvoir put it, to coincide with yourself.

LIST OF ILLUSTRATIONS

p. xvi
Advertisement for Iodamelis, from the Laboratoires Jacques Logeais 71, Avenue de Clamart, Issy-les-Moulineaux, Paris.
Wellcome Library, London

p. 71
Engraving by Jeremias Falck after a Johann Liss painting which formed part of the Dutch Gift to Charles II in 1660.
Wellcome Library, London

p. 80
French wax figure, *c.* 1760, by Anara Morandi Mazzolini of Bologna.
Wellcome Library, London

p. 106
Plate from Alexander Walker's *Beauty: Illustrated Chiefly by an Analysis and Classification of Beauty in Woman* (London, 1836).
Wellcome Library, London

p. 153
Cartoon by Félicien Rops (1800–1899).
Wellcome Library, London

p. 202
Advertisement for Endocreme from *Life* magazine, May 3 1948.

NOTES

Introduction

1 Stolberg, M., 'A woman's hell? Medical perceptions of menopause in preindustrial Europe' in *Bulletin of the History of Medicine* (1999), 73, 404–28.

2 In the UK in the 1960s there was a sustained 'baby boom' when births rose to a peak of 1,014,700 in 1964 (2.95 children per woman); this was followed by a rapid decline until a low of 657,000 was reached in 1977. Numbers of births rose again in the late 1980s and early 1990s, the result of the large number of female 'baby boomers', and in 2005 there were over 722,500 births (1.79 children per woman).

3 International Menopause Society, see www.imsociety.org

4 Ferguson, S. J. and Parry, C., 'Rewriting menopause: Challenging the medical paradigm to reflect menopausal women's experiences' in *Frontiers: A Journal of Women's Studies*, 19 (1) (1998), 20–41.

5 Hormone replacement therapy (HRT) is, briefly, the provision of oestrogen (with progesterone in women who have hung on to their uterus).

6 Double standards are plain in our divergent attitudes to men and women who come late to parenthood, witness the difference in attitudes to fathers in their fifties and older who are celebrated and the vilification of women who become mothers at that age. It isn't the case that all the risks revolve around an older mother: men over forty are six times more likely to father a child with autism than their younger peers and risk rises steadily with advancing age.

7 Pelling, R., 'Watch out boys – Jan is the future. Sexy, sixty and single. Today's older ladies will not keep their sexuality quiet. Lock up your sons . . .' in the *Independent on Sunday*, 26 November 2006.

8 Feinson, M. C., 'Where are women in the history of aging?' in *Social Science History*, 9 (4) (Fall 1985), 429–52, 448, fn 9.

9 Cherry, K., et al., review of Gullette, M., *Aged by Culture* in *Biography*, 27 (3) (Summer 2004), 631–4.

10 Sontag, S., 'The double standard of ageing' in Carver, V., and Liddiard, P. (eds.), *An Ageing Population* (London: Hodder and Stoughton, OUP, 1978).

11 Steinem, G., *Revolution from Within: A Book of Self-Esteem* (London: Bloomsbury, 1992), pp. 244, 246.

12 Fothergill, J., *Of the management proper at the cessation of the menses* (London, 1774).

1   The Modern Menopause

1 Marinello, G., *Le medicine partenenti alle infermità delle donne* (Venice, 1563); Wilson, R. A., *Feminine Forever* (London: WH Allen, 1966).

2 Stolberg, M., 'A woman's hell? Medical perceptions of menopause in preindustrial Europe' in *Bulletin of the History of Medicine* (1999), 73, 404–28, 404.

3 Kirkwood, T., *Time of Our Lives: The Science of Human Ageing* (London: Weidenfield and Nicolson, 1999), p. 166; te Velde, E. R., 'Concepts in female reproductive ageing' in te Velde, E. R., Pearson, P. L., and Broekmans, F. J. (eds.), *Female Reproductive Aging. Studies in Profertility Series Vol. 9. The Proceedings of the 10th Reinier de Graaf Symposium, Zeist, The Netherlands, 9–11 September 1999* (London: Parthenon Publishing Group, 2000), pp. 49–57.

4 Macklon, N. S., and Fauser, B. C. J. M., 'Follicle development before and during the menstrual cycle' in te Velde, et al., pp. 111–22.

5 Walton, J., Beeson, P. B., and Bodley Scott, R. (eds), *The Oxford Companion to Medicine* (Oxford: OUP, 1986), vol. 1, p. 339.

6 The gonads, in humans, are the ovary in the female and the testis in the male, and gonadotrophin is one of the hormones which controls their function.

7 Baird, D. T., 'The ovary' in Austin, C. R., and Short, R. V., *Reproduction in Mammals. Book 3: Hormonal Control of Reproduction* (Cambridge: CUP, 2nd edn., 1984), ch. 5, pp. 91–114.

8 Lambalk, C. B., Van Montfraus, J. M., and de Koning, C. H., 'Clinical consequences of elevated follicle stimulating hormone levels in the patient treated for infertility' in te Velde, et al., pp. 249–60.

9 Hunt, P. A., 'The control of mammalian female meiosis and the factors that influence chromosome segregation' in te Velde, et al., pp. 185–96.

10 Berger, G. E., *Menopause and Culture* (London: Pluto, 1999), pp. 2–3.

11 Dillaway, H. E., 'When does menopause occur, and how long does it

last.' Wrestling with age- and time-based conceptualizations of reproductive aging' in *NWSA Journal*, 18 (1) (Spring 2006), 31–61.

12 Judd, H. L., 'The basis of menopausal vasomotor symptoms' in Mastroianni, L., and Paulsen, C. A. (eds.), *Aging, Reproduction, and the Climacteric* (New York: Plenum Press, 1986), pp. 215–28.

13 Ibid., pp. 2, 4; Greer, G., *The Change: Women, Ageing and the Menopause* (London: Hamish Hamilton, 1991), p. 112; Murray, J., *Is it Me or is it Hot in Here? A Modern Woman's Guide to Menopause* (London: Vermilion, 2001), p. 11.

14 Murray, p. 17.

15 Gold, J. M., *The Psychiatric Implications of Menstruation* (Washington, DC: American Psychiatric Press Inc., 1986), p. 99.

16 Gannon, L. R., *Women and Aging: Transcending the Myths* (London: Routledge, 1999).

17 The UK Department of Health estimates that *c.* 85,000 people fracture a hip each year, and about nineteen in twenty of these are the result of falls suffered by people with osteoporosis. Taking 1000 mg of calcium each day (a pint of milk or 2 oz of hard cheese) can reduce the risk of hip fractures.

18 The World Health Organization (WHO) identifies osteoporosis as a priority health issue and classifies it with other major non-communicable diseases. In Europe the annual costs associated with osteoporotic fractures is estimated as *c.* €25 billion, and in the UK at over £1.7 billion per year.

19 http://www.nos.org.uk

20 According to the Royal College of Psychiatry, British girls and women are ten times more likely than boys and men to suffer from anorexia or bulimia. About 1 in 200 women and 1 in 2000 men become anorexic at some time in their lives, and about 4 out of every 100 women suffers from bulimia at some point; fewer men suffer, though eating disorders seem to be getting more common in boys and men. In America the National Association of Anorexia Nervosa and Associated Disorders (ANAD) states that approximately 8 million people, that is *c.* 3 per cent, in the US have anorexia nervosa, bulimia and related eating disorders; males make up *c.* 10 per cent of these. As American 'baby boomers' grow older, there seems to be an increase in the incidence of middle-aged women with anorexia and bulimia. Researchers also believe that whilst the prevalence of eating disorders in non-Western countries is lower than that of Western countries, it appears to be increasing.

21 Kirby, J., 'Cola linked to brittle bones' in the *Independent*, 6 October 2006. A recent American study has suggested that if a woman drinks just four cans of cola or diet cola a week it could lead to brittle bones. It found that the risk of lower bone mineral density, and therefore of osteoporosis, in women's hips, was increased, regardless of age, timing of menopause, calcium and vitamin D intake, smoking or drinking alcohol. Where previous studies have suggested that findings were due to cola replacing milk in the diet, in this study the women drinking cola had the same milk intake as those who were not. Argument continues as to the effects of a regular intake of phosphoric acid found in colas. Drinking cola was not associated with lower bone mineral density in men.

22 Abbott, E., *A History of Celibacy* (Cambridge: Butterworth Press, 2001), pp. 299–300.

23 Fordney, D. S., 'Female sexuality during and following menopause' in Mastroianni and Paulsen, pp. 229–40.

24 Ibid., p. 229. Sexual dysfunction in men over forty (erectile failure being categorized as the most significant characteristic) is attributed to physiology, whereas the 'reality probably rests somewhere in between for both sexes'.

25 Kinsey, A. C., *Sexual Behavior in the Human Female* (Philadelphia: Saunders, 1953), pp. 353–4.

26 Berger, p. 4.

27 Basson, R., et al., 'Revised definitions of women's sexual dysfunction' in *The Journal of Sexual Medicine*, 1 (July 2004), 40.

28 Goldstein, I., and Alexander, J. L., 'Practical aspects in the management of vaginal atrophy and sexual dysfunction in perimenopausal and postmenopausal women' in *The Journal of Sexual Medicine*, 2 (September 2005), 154.

29 www.studd.co.uk

30 Department of Health Prodigy Guidance, www.prodigy.nhs.uk

01 Davis, S. R., et al., 'Endocrine aspects of female sexual dysfunction' in *The Journal of Sexual Medicine*, 1 (July 2004), 82.

32 Dennerstein, L., and Hayes, R. D., 'Confronting the challenges: Epidemiological study of female sexual dysfunction and the menopause' in *The Journal of Sexual Medicine*, 2 (September 2005), 118.

33 Winterich, J. A., 'Sex, menopause, and culture: Sexual orientation and the meaning of menopause for women's sex lives' in *Gender & Society*, 17 (4) (August 2003), 627–42.

34 Ibid.

35 *Observer*, 14 May 2006.

36 These IUDs are effective long-term so are recommended for women over the age of thirty-five who are more concerned with having no more pregnancies than with spacing them out; the IUD can be left in place until menopause is established. There is a low incidence of side-effects, including bleeding and infection. According to a WHO Scientific Group on the Menopause the levonorgestrel-releasing IUD, which has a local suppressive effect on the endometrium by releasing constant low levels of progestogen, is even more suitable for 'late premenopausal years' due to 'high acceptability [and] minimal bleeding problems', thus its use as a treatment for menorrhagia (abnormally heavy menstrual flow).

37 Diaphragms and condoms are the most common barrier methods but they are less effective than IUDs or the pill, though they do offer protection against sexually transmitted diseases. The WHO believes they are suitable for menopausal women because fecundity is low, which is true enough, but they also seem to believe that 'the frequency of coitus [is] low' too, which may take some of you by surprise.

38 Types of contraceptive pill currently on the market have four to five times less oestrogen and progestogen in them than those on offer in the 1960s following studies in the 1970s and 80s that revealed health risks in the original high-dose preparations. In women over thirty-five there is a slight increase in risk of stroke through use of current combined oral contraceptives, and smoking and high blood pressure increase this risk. There is a slight increase in risk of venous thromboembolism which becomes apparent in the first few months of taking the pill and disappears in the few months after stopping. The increased risk of breast cancer during and after the menopause would be exacerbated by taking the pill – it 'would be a significant problem'. Progestogen-only pills might be recommended for women who are at risk of cardiovascular disease but these drugs are less effective.

39 Kirkwood, p. 168.

40 Sample, I., 'Gene mutation test predicts likelihood of early menopause' in the *Guardian*, 7 February 2006.

41 Smoking has long been associated with early-onset menopause. The habit has been shown to have a profound effect on FSH levels which signal the onset of menopausal transition and affect fertility. Concentrations of FSH have been found to be 66 per cent higher in

active smokers and 39 per cent higher in passive smokers compared with controls. See te Velde, et al., p. 255.

42 Women born in the UK in 1943 had their first child at the average age of 23.8 years. Those born in 1959, the most recent cohort to have reached the end of their child-bearing years, had their first child at the average age of 25.7 years. In 2005 the average age of women having their first birth was 27.3 years, a rise of 3.6 years from 1970, and 2.8 years from 1960. About one in five women in their mid-forties in 2005, born around 1960, were childless, compared with one in ten women born in the mid-1940s, who were childless at the same age. In America, over the last three decades, the average age of mothers at first birth has shifted steadily upwards from 24.6 years to 27.2 years. According to the National Center for Health Statistics this trend in delayed childbirth has been observed nationwide and among all population groups (yet with variations by state and by race). The number of women going through college since 1970 has nearly doubled, as has the number in the labour force.

43 Apter, T., *Secret Paths: Women in the New Midlife* (London: W.W. Norton & Company, 1995), pp. 215, 216.

44 McKinlay, J. B., and McKinlay, S. M., 'Depression in middle-aged women: Social circumstances versus estrogen deficiency' in Walsh, M. R., *The Psychology of Women* (New Haven: Yale University Press, 1987), pp. 157–61.

45 Nicol-Smith, L., 'Causality, menopause, and depression: A critical review of the literature', *BMJ* (1996), 313 (1067), 1229–32.

46 Hunter, M. S., 'Depression and menopause', *BMJ* (1996), 313 (1067), 1217–18.

47 Carey, B., 'A rhythm to women's blues' in *Health* (1996), 10 (5), 23; Woods, N. F., et al., 'Patterns of depressed mood in midlife women: Observations from the Seattle Women's Health Study' in *Research in Nursing and Health* (1996), 19 (2), 111–23.

48 Apter, pp. 201–7.

49 Kirkwood, pp. 163, 167, 169. Professor Kirkwood gave the 2001 Reith Lectures on 'The End of Age' and is Britain's first Professor of Biological Gerontology at the University of Manchester and now Professor of Medicine and Head of the Department of Gerontology at the University of Newcastle.

50 Gosden, R. G., and Finch, C. E., 'Definition and character of reproductive aging and senescence', in te Velde, et al., pp. 11–25. In what are

called 'natural fertility' societies, such as the North American Hutterites, the decline in fertility begins in the middle of the fourth decade and c. 50 per cent of married women have had their last child at forty, ten years before the menopause.

51 Kirkwood, T., 'Similarities of general reproductive ageing', pp. 43–7, in te Velde, et al., pp. 46–7. Kirkwood suggests that one possible reason for neurons lasting longer is that 'quality assurance' on eggs necessarily needs to be so much more rigorous.

52 Kirkwood, *Time of Our Lives*, p. 170. He gives the example of traditional West African societies in which post-menopausal women are liberated from the restrictions associated with child-bearing women and attain a higher status within their communities.

53 Hawkes, R., O'Connell, J. F., and Blurton-Jones, N. G., 'Why do women have a mid-life menopause? Grandmothering and the evolution of human longevity' in te Velde, et al., pp. 27–41.

54 Cant, M. A., and Johnstone, R. A., 'Reproductive conflict and the separation of reproductive generations in humans' in *PNAS*, 31 March 2008.

55 Kirkwood, p. 171. To compare, Kirkwood cites an anthropological study of the Ache people of the eastern Paraguay rainforest which shows that, despite high infant mortality, six out of ten females survive to the average age of first birth (between nineteen and twenty years) and they then have a further life expectancy of about forty years, which means that they experience the menopause.

56 A very gracious, not to mention serene, acronym – an 'appropriate' creation some might say . . .

57 Avis, N., et al., 'Is there a menopausal syndrome? Menopausal status and symptoms across racial/ethnic groups' in *Social Science & Medicine* (2001), 52, 345–56. In India, for example, women of the Rajput caste have few problems in menopause apart from cycle changes, reporting no depression, dizziness or other incapacitation. Only a small proportion of Japanese women aged 45–55 years experience depression or irritability and these symptoms vary little with menopausal status.

58 Coney, S., *The Menopause Industry* (London: Women's Press, 1995).

59 MacPherson, K., 'Going to the source: Women reclaim menopause' in *Feminist Studies*, 21 (2) (Summer 1995), 347.

60 Ferguson, S. J., and Parry, C., 'Rewriting menopause: Challenging the medical paradigm to reflect menopausal women's experiences' in *Frontiers: A Journal of Women's Studies*, 19 (1) (1998), 35.

61 Moscucci, O., *The Science of Women: Gynaecology and Gender in England, 1800–1929* (Cambridge: CUP, 1990), pp. 1–2. Moscucci ponders whether it is conceivable that the rationale for differentiating the medical specialism of gynaecology, as it is at present, may one day cease to exist, p. 6.

62 Flemming, R., *Medicine and the Making of Roman Women: Gender, Nature, and Authority from Celsus to Galen* (Oxford: OUP, 2000), pp. 4–6, 22, 25, 26.

63 Porter, R., *The Cambridge Illustrated History of Medicine* (Cambridge: CUP, 1996), p. 110.

64 Szasz, T., *The Myth of Mental Illness: Foundations of a Theory of Personal Conduct* (London: Secker & Warburg, 1962).

65 Greenblatt, R. B., and Teran, A-Z., 'Advice to post-menopausal women' in Zichella, L., Whitehead, M. I., and van Keep, P. A. (eds.), *The Climacteric and Beyond* (Proceedings of the 5th International Congress on the Menopause 1987 . . . under the auspices of the International Menopause Society), ch. 4, pp. 39–53. Robert Greenblatt (1907–87) was Professor Emeritus of Endocrinology at the Medical College of Georgia, USA.

66 Apter, pp. 210–11.

2   Bad Blood and Beasts

1 Skinner, H. A., *The Origin of Medical Terms* (Baltimore: Williams & Wilkins, 1970). From Greek *klimakterikos*, a critical event or period, from *klimakter*, a rung of a ladder, from *klimax*, a ladder + *-ikos* of, relating to, or resembling.

2 Dean-Jones, L., *Women's Bodies in Classical Greek Science* (Oxford: OUP, 1994), p. 108; Flemming, R., *Medicine and the Making of Roman Women: Gender, Nature, and Authority from Celsus to Galen* (Oxford: OUP), pp. 117, 120. In Pliny's account the womb is a body apart, an addition to the main, male body.

3 Dean-Jones, pp. 105–8.

4 Was, indeed, gynaecology actually necessary? Helen King, 'gynaecology', *The Oxford Classical Dictionary*, ed. Simon Hornblower and Anthony Spawforth (Oxford: OUP, 2003). *Oxford Reference Online* – <http://www.oxfordreference.com/views/ENTRY.html?subview=Main&entry=t111.e2909>

5 Hippocrates, born at Cos, was educated by the followers of Aesculapius who formed an organized guild of physicians. Temples dedicated to him became sanitaria and were run by priest-physicians; medicine was also practised and studied by the philosophers and the gymnasts. See

Medvei, V. C., *A History of Endocrinology* (Lancaster, UK: MTP Press Ltd, 1982), p. 40.

6 Hankinson, R. J. (ed.), *Galen* (Cambridge: CUP, 2008).

7 Dean-Jones, p. 26.

8 Ibid., pp. 6–7, 10.

9 Schiebinger, L. 'Mammals, primatology and sexology' in Porter, R., and Teich, M. (eds.), *Sexual Knowledge, Sexual Science: A History of Attitudes to Sexuality* (Cambridge: CUP, 1994), pp. 110–12.

10 Dean-Jones, pp. 246–7. Many priesstesshoods seem to have been reserved for post-menopausal women. Plutarch says that the Pythia was the only woman allowed in the temple at Delphi and that she had to be past fifty years old.

11 Nutton, V., in Porter, R., *The Cambridge History of Medicine* (Cambridge: CUP, 1996), pp. 52-81.

12 Crawford, P., 'Attitudes to menstruation in seventeenth-century England', in *Past & Present*, 91 (May 1981), 47–73.

13 King, H., 'Bound to bleed: Artemis and Greek women' in Cameron, A., and Kuhrt, A. (eds.), *Images of Women in Antiquity* (London: Routledge, 1991), pp. 109–27.

14 Dean-Jones, pp. 20–1, 85.

15 Schiebinger in Porter and Teich (eds.), pp. 184–209. Galen uses the term 'horns' to describe the Fallopian tubes, which could be said to protrude from the womb in such a fashion; the Hippocratics, however, show no knowledge of these; see Dean-Jones, pp. 66–7.

16 Flemming, p. 117.

17 Ibid., p. 311. 'The hair of the beard not only protects the jaws but also contributes to their seemliness: for the male seems more august, especially as he grows older, if he has everywhere a good covering of hair. On this account also nature has left the so-called 'apples' (cheeks) and nose smooth and bare of hair; for otherwise the whole countenance would have become savage and bestial, by no means suitable for a civilised and social animal . . . On the other hand, for women, the rest of whose body is always soft and hairless like a child's, the bareness of the face would not be unseemly, and besides, this animal does not have an august character as the man has and so does not need an august form. For I have already shown many times, if not throughout the work, that nature makes the form of the body appropriate to the characteristics of the soul. And the female genus does not need any special covering as protection against the cold, since for the most part women

stay at home, yet they do need long hair on their heads, for both protection and seemliness, and this they share with men', pp. 320–1.

18 Eadie, M. J., and Bladin, P. F., *A Disease Once Sacred: A History of the Medical Understanding of Epilepsy* (Eastleigh: John Libbey & Co. Ltd, 2001), p. 71.

19 Flemming, pp. 333–4.

20 Dean-Jones, pp. 105–8.

21 Ibid., pp. 27, 105–8, 134–5, 182–3.

22 Chadwick, H., 'Christian doctrine' in Burns, J. H. (ed.), *The Cambridge History of Medieval Political Thought c. 350–c. 1450* (Cambridge: CUP, 1991), p. 16.

23 Crawford, pp. 49, 57.

24 Meacham, T., 'An abbreviated history of the development of the Jewish menstrual laws' in Wasserfall, R. (ed.), *Women and Water: Menstruation in Jewish Life and Law* (Hanover, New Hampshire: University Press of New England, 1999), pp. 23–39.

25 Amundsen, D. W., and Diers, C. J., 'The age of menopause in medieval Europe' in *Human Biology*, 45 (4) (December 1973), 605–12.

26 Amundsen and Diers, pp. 606–9.

27 Post, J. B., 'Ages at menarche and menopause: Some mediaeval authorities' in *Population Studies* (1971), xxv, 83–7.

28 Crawford, p. 49.

29 Ibid., p. 54.

30 The term 'flowers' was commonly used for the menses because, just as trees without their flowers cannot bear fruit, neither can women without theirs bear children, in Green, M. (ed., trans.), *The Trotula: A Mediaeval Compendium of Women's Medicine* (Philadelphia: University of Pennsylvania Press, 2001), p. 21.

31 Stolberg, M., 'A woman's hell? Medical perceptions of menopause in preindustrial Europe' in *Bulletin of the History of Medicine* (1999), 73, 407–15.

32 Fontaine, N., *The Womans Doctour or, an exact and distinct Explanation of all such Diseases as peculiar to that Sex. With Choice and Experimentall Remedies against the same* (London, 1652), p. 71.

33 Crawford, P., 'Attitudes to menstruation in seventeenth-century England' in *Past and Present*, 91 (May 1981), 56–7.

34 Nutton, p. 23. Fontaine, p. 112. Fanny Burney (1752–1840) gave a detailed account of her mastectomy, performed in 1811, which is included in ch. 3.

35 Fontaine, pp. 112, 116–17.

36 Manning, H., *A Treatise of Female Diseases* (London: printed for R. Baldwin, 1771), pp. 60–2.

37 *Bancke's Herbal*, p. 44; see also Hill, J., Brightly, C., and Kinnersley, T., *The Family Herbal* (Bungay: C. Brightly & Co., 1812), p. 237, and Trovillion, V. and H., *Recipes and Remedies of Early England* (Herrin, Ill.: Trovillion Private Press, 1946). The herb appears in a recent work by Crawford, A. M., *The Herbal Menopause Book* (Berkeley: The Crossing Press, 1996), p. 162.

38 Fontaine, p. 1. He was moved to write his book from a 'need to correct [the] inconvenience' of fellow physicians who may have read a rival's book and could 'sooner finde your Patient dead, than a remedy in his writings for her recovery'.

39 Crawford, pp. 56, 66–7 fn 114, 71.

40 Rowland, B., *Medieval Woman's Guide to Health: The First English Gynecological Handbook* (London: Croom Helm, 1981), p. 59.

41 Ibid., pp. 61, 67.

42 Ehrenreich, B., and English, D., *For Her Own Good: 150 Years of the Expert's Advice to Women* (London: Pluto Press, 1979), p. 32.

43 Amundsen and Diers, pp. 607–8.

44 Nutton, in Porter (ed.), *The Cambridge Illustrated History of Medicine*, p. 80. In *c.* 1413–15 Kempe left on her great pilgrimages via Norwich, Great Yarmouth, Zierikzee, Constance, Bologna, Venice, the Holy Land, Venice, Assisi, Rome, Middelburg and Norwich. In *c.* 1417–18 she travelled through England and Spain and in 1433 she went to Prussia and back. See Goodman, A., *Margery Kempe and her World* (London: Pearson Education Ltd, 2002).

45 Rowland, p. 59.

46 Sadler, J., *The Sicke Womans Private Looking-Glasse wherein Methodically are handled all uterine affects, or diseases arising from the Wombe; enabling Women to informe the Physician about the cause of their griefe* . . . (London: printed by Anne Griffin for Philemon Stephens and Christopher Meredith, 1636).

47 Crawford, P., 'Sexual knowledge in England 1500–1750' in Porter, R., and Teich, M. (eds.), *Sexual Knowledge, Sexual Science: A History of Attitudes to Sexuality* (Cambridge: CUP, 1994), pp. 82–106. Even by the late eighteenth to late nineteenth centuries the rise of the man-midwife came in for some vicious condemnation like this. Frank Nicholls thought male midwives allowed 'to treat our wives in such a manner . . . frequently ends in their destruction, and to have such intercourse with our women, as easily shifts into indecency, from indecency into obscenity, and from obscenity into debauchery'. George Morant in *Hints to Husbands*

(1857) thought women were 'invaded *by the presence, and violated by the actual contact* of the *man*-midwife'. It was unspeakable 'scientific' rascaldom, hypocritically masquerading as scientific discovery. A violation of women, a challenge to men. Moscucci, O., *The Science of Women: Gynaecology and Gender in England, 1800–1929* (Cambridge: CUP, 1990), p. 118.

48 Garcia-Ballester, L., et al., 'Documenting medieval women's medical practice' in Green, M. (ed.), *Women's Health Care in the Medieval West* (Aldershot: Ashgate Publishing Ltd, 2000), pp. 322–52. Nutton, p. 76.

49 Ehrenreich and English, *For Her Own Good*, p. 32.

50 'Obstetrical and gynaecological texts in Middle English' in Green, *Women's Health Care in the Medieval West*, pp. 53–88.

51 The physician to Edward II, who had a degree in theology and a doctorate in medicine from Oxford, prescribed for the toothache writing on the jaw of the patient 'In the name of the Father, the Son, and the Holy Ghost, Amen', and this when witches were being persecuted and burnt. In America medical practice was generally open to anybody who could demonstrate healing skills and the tradition of female lay healing flourished in colonial America and the early republic, combining as it did all the knowledge from the old countries plus the knowledge and skills of the Native Americans. The North American female healer was not eliminated by violence, like her European sisters, but by economics and the growth of the medical marketplace as the healing business as it was separated from the community and personal relationships. Ehrenreich and English, *For Her Own Good*, pp. 33–6.

52 Stolberg, pp. 404–28.

53 Trevor-Roper, H. R., *The European Witch-Craze of the Sixteenth and Seventeenth Century* (London: Penguin Books, 1990), p. 15.

54 The original Hebrew is more accurately translated as 'Thou shalt not suffer a poisoner to live.' Being obsessed with witchcraft, James VI had deliberately mis-translated the original text. He also wrote *Demonologie*, a famous learned treatise on the subject, in 1597.

55 Heinemann, E., *Witches: A Psychoanalytic Exploration of the Killing of Women*, trans. Kiraly, D. (London: Free Association Books, 2000), p. 19.

56 Stolberg, p. 416.

57 Groneman, C., 'Nymphomania: The historical construction of female sexuality' in *Signs: Journal of Women in Culture and Society*, 19, (2), 341.

58 Heinemann, p. 18.

59 Hufton, O., *The Prospect Before Her: A History of Women in Western Europe*,

Volume 1, 1500–1800 (London: HarperCollins, 1995), p. 480. It has been argued that the excuse of hormonal imbalance as a mitigating factor in deviant behaviour should not be a political issue as modern medicine can control other more serious hormonal illnesses, such as diabetes and Addison's disease – which sounds as though the suggestion is for women to medicate themselves for life to avoid 'deviance'. Dean-Jones, p. 253.

60 Larner, C., *Witchcraft and Religion: The Politics of Popular Belief* (Oxford: Blackwell, 1984), *passim*.

61 Fear of the aggression of declining families is a characteristic of peasant societies. See Foster, G., 'Peasant society and the image of a limited good' in *American Anthropologist* (1965), 67 (2), 302.

62 Holmes, R., *Coleridge: Early Visions* (London: Penguin Books, 1990), p. 215.

63 During the Laudian reforms and antipathy to Puritanism of the 1630s, Essex, in England, saw one of the largest emigrations of clergy and laity of all the counties to New England – an emigration that had its dire repercussions in Salem.

64 Godbeer, R., *The Devil's Dominion: Magic and Religion in Early New England* (Cambridge: CUP, 1992).

65 Trevor-Roper, pp. 8–9, 15. In the fifty years between 1580 and 1630, for instance, the witch-craze corresponded with the mature life of Bacon and brought together figures such as Montaigne and Descartes.

66 Heinemann, pp. 18–20.

67 Ibid.; Green, *The Trotula*, p. 20.

68 St Clair, W., and Maassen, I. (eds.), *Conduct Literature for Women 1500–1640*, (London: Pickering & Chatto, c. 2000), vol. 2, p. 324.

69 Ibid., vol. 6, pp. 293–4. He did also admit that 'the like may be said of our stale Batchelors'.

70 Pennell, S. (ed.), *Women in Medicine: Remedy Books, 1533–1865* (Wellcome Library, London, Primary Source Microfilm). The books, kept by all manner of women from alchemists to aristocrats, hold a narrative of their lives: one contains recipe after recipe 'to prevent miscarriage' which are nearly all annotated with the deeply poignant phrase 'not found to be effective'.

71 Woolley, H., *The Gentlewoman's Companion . . .* (London: printed by A. Maxwell for Edward Thomas, 1675), pp. 44–6, 61, 174, 178. For a top and tail the gentlewoman might continue with a remedy 'Against Kibed Heels . . . Make a hole in the top of a Turnip, take out some of the pith, & pour into the hole oyl of Roses, then stop the hole close, and roast it

under hot Embers; when it is soft, apply it Plaister-wise to the Kibe as hot as can be endured.'

72 Gatrell, V. A. C., *City of Laughter: Sex and Satire in Fighteenth-Century London* (London: Atlantic Books, 2006). Professor Gatrell notes Freud's view of misogynistic humour as arising from a threat to a man's libidinal impulse, a 'hostile trend' against women, and the joke shared with a male ally.

73 Ibid., pp. 345–6.

3   Their Nature Explained

1 Medvei, V. C., *A History of Endocrinology* (Lancaster, UK: MTP Press Ltd, 1982), pp. 19, 106. It has been said that Herophilos described the ovaries in the third century BC. The ancient Egyptians are reputed to have performed ovariotomies for the purpose of contraception. Walton, J., Beeson, Paul B., and Bodley Scott, R. (eds.), *The Oxford Companion to Medicine* (Oxford: OUP, 1986), vol. 1, p. 337.

2 Medvei, p. 118.

3 te Velde, E. R., 'Preface: Reinier de Graaf and his symposium' in te Velde, E. R., Pearson, P. L., and Brockmans, F. J. (eds.), *Female Reproductive Aging* (London: Parthenon Publishing Group, 2000), pp. xiii–xvi.

4 Ibid.

5 Adams, J., *Observations on Morbid Poisons, Phagedena, and Cancer* (London, 1795), p. 176, quoted in Shorter, E., *A History of Women's Bodies* (London: Allen Lane, 1983), p. 68.

6 Smellie, W., *A Treatise on the Theory and Practice of Midwifery* (1752); *Oxford Dictionary of National Biography* (Oxford: OUP, 2004–6).

7 Anderson, J. (c. 1730–1804), *Medical Remarks on Natural, Spontaneous and Artificial Evacuation* (London: printed for the author and sold by J. Murray and by J. Donaldson, Edinburgh, 1787), pp. 78, 81.

8 Freind, John, *Emmenologia* (London: Thomas Bennet, 1703), pp. 61–2.

9 Lord, A., 'The great *Arcana* of the deity: Menstruation and menstrual disorders in eighteenth-century British medical thought' in *Bulletin of the History of Medicine*, 73 (1) (Spring 1999), pp. 38–63.

10 Moscucci, O., *The Science of Women: Gynaecology and Gender in England, 1800–1929* (Cambridge: CUP, 1990), pp. 10–12.

11 Lord, p. 40.

12 Moscucci, p. 13.

13 Leake, J., *Medical Instructions Towards the Prevention and Cure of Chronic or Slow Diseases Peculiar to Women: Especially those proceeding from over-delicacy of habit called Nervous or Hysterical; from Female Obstructions, Weakness and inward Decay; a*

diseased state of the Womb, or critical Change of Constitution at particular Periods of Life, in which, their Nature is explained, and their Treatment by Regimen, and simple Medicines . . . (London: printed for R. Baldwin, 1777), p. 85.

14 Astruc, J. (1684–1766), *A Treatise on all the Diseases Incident to Women* (London: S. Highley, 1844), p. 57; Leake, pp. 84–5.

15 Manning, H., *A Treatise of Female Diseases* (London: printed for R. Baldwin, 1771), pp. 57–9, 362–5.

16 Porter, R., *Mind-Forg'd Manacles: A History of Madness in England from the Restoration to the Regency* (London: Penguin Books, 1990), pp. 105–8.

17 Leake, pp. 9, 12, 16, 37, 43, 86–8.

18 Manning, p. 58; Leake, pp. 85, 89, 92.

19 Foxcroft, L., *The Making of Addiction: The Use and Abuse of Opiates in Nineteenth-Century Britain* (Aldershot: Ashgate Publishing Ltd, 2007).

20 DeLacy, M., 'Fothergill, John (1712–1780), physician and naturalist' in *Oxford Dictionary of National Biography*.

21 Stolberg, M., 'A woman's hell? Medical perceptions of menopause in preindustrial Europe' in *Bulletin of the History of Medicine* (1999), 73, 414.

22 Wilbush, J., 'Climacteric disorders – historical perspectives' in Studd, J. W. W., and Whitehead, M. I. (eds.), *The Menopause* (Oxford: Blackwell Scientific Publications, 1988), pp. 1–14.

23 Rousseau, J-J., *Emile*, trans. Foxley, B. (London: Dent, 1974), p. 218.

24 Stolberg, pp. 416–17.

25 Ibid., pp. 423–4.

26 Ibid., pp. 421–2; Bell, S. G., and Offen, K. M. (eds.), *Women, the Family, and Freedom: The Debate in Documents, Vol. 1: 1750–1880* (Stanford: Stanford University Press, 1983).

27 Shorter, E., *A History of Women's Bodies* (London: Penguin, 1983), pp. 245–6.

28 Shorter, E., 'Women's diseases before 1900' in Albin, M. (ed.), with the assistance of Devlin, R. J., and Heeger, G., *New Directions in Psychohistory: The Adelphi Papers in Honor of Erik H. Erikson* (London: Allen Lane, 1983), ch. 13, pp. 183–208.

4   On the Borderland of Pathology

1 Shaw, S., 'Spontaneous combustion and the sectioning of female bodies' in *Literature and Medicine*, 14 (1) (Spring 1995), 1–22.

2 Shaw, *passim*.

3 Charles Dickens, in his preface to *Bleak House* (London: Penguin Books, 1996), pp. 6–7.

4 Gatrell, V. A., *City of Laughter: Sex and Satire in Eighteenth-Century London* (London: Atlantic Books, 2006), pp. 346, 354.

5 Moscucci, O., *The Science of Women: Gynaecology and Gender in England, 1800–1929* (Cambridge: CUP, 1990), pp. 35–6.

6 Ripa, Y. (trans.), Catherine du Peloux Menagé, *Women and Madness: The Incarceration of Women in Nineteenth-Century France* (Cambridge: Polity Press, 1990), p. 51.

7 Walker, A., *Beauty: Illustrated Chiefly by an Analysis and Classification of Beauty in Woman* (London: E. Wilson, 1836), pp. 170, 173, 177.

8 Ibid., p. 70.

9 Featherstone, M., and Hepworth, M., 'The history of the male menopause 1848–1936' in *Maturitas* (1985), 7, 250.

10 Ibid.

11 Stedman, J., 'From dame to woman: W. S. Gilbert and theatrical transvestism' in Vicinus, M. (ed.), *Suffer and Be Still: Women in the Victorian Age* (Bloomington: Indiana University Press, 1972), pp. 20–37.

12 Stewart, M. L., *For Health and Beauty: Physical Culture for Frenchwomen, 1880s–1930s* (Baltimore: The Johns Hopkins University Press, 2001), p. 131.

13 Orr, L., *Jules Michelet: Nature, History, and Language* (Ithaca: Cornell University Press, 1976), p. 3.

14 Marañón, G., trans. Stevens, K. S., *The Climacteric (The Critical Age)* (St Louis: C. V. Mosby, 1929). The work was first published in Spain in 1925, then across Europe and in America.

15 *Lancet*, 367, 20 May 2006, 1647–8.

16 Porter, R., *Mind-Forg'd Manacles: A History of Madness in England from the Restoration to the Regency* (London: Penguin Books, 1990), p. 44.

17 Michel Foucault, in *The History of Sexuality*, vol. 1, p. 104, terms this the 'hysterization of women's bodies' and describes a 'threefold process whereby the feminine body was analyzed – qualified and disqualified – as being thoroughly saturated with sexuality; whereby it was integrated into the sphere of medical practice, by reason of a pathology intrinsic to it; whereby it was placed in organic communication with the social body . . . the family space . . . and the life of children'.

18 See, for example, Walkowitz, J. R., *Prostitution and Victorian Society: Women, Class, and the State* (Cambridge: CUP, 1980) on the response to the Contagious Diseases Acts in the 1860s.

19 Vertinsky, P., *The Eternally Wounded Woman: Women, Doctors and Exercise in the Late Nineteenth Century* (Manchester: Manchester University Press, 1990), pp. 89–95.

20 Menville de Ponsan, C., *De l'âge critique chez les femmes: des maladies qui peuvent*

survenir à cette époque de la vie, et des moyens de les combattre et de les prévenir (Paris, 1840).

21 Corfe, G., *Man and His Many Changes or, Seven Times Seven* (London: Houlston and Wright, 1849), p. 73.

22 Ashwell, S., *Practical Treatise on the Diseases Peculiar to Women* (London: S. Highley, 1844), pp. 196–201. Ashwell was a member of the Royal College of Physicians and obstetric physician and lecturer at Guy's Hospital, London.

23 Porter, R., *The Cambridge Illustrated History of Medicine* (Cambridge: CUP), pp. 96–7.

24 Mason, S., *The Turn of Life* (1845).

25 Anderson, O., *Suicide in Victorian and Edwardian England* (Oxford: Clarendon Press, 1987).

26 Marañón, p. 222.

27 Moscucci, p. 36.

28 Tilt, E. J., *The Change of Life in Health and Disease. A Practical Treatise on the Nervous and Other Affections Incidental to Women at the Decline of Life* (London: John Churchill, 1857).

29 Compton Burnett, J., *The Change of Life in Women and the Ills and Ailings Incident Thereto* (London: The Homeopathic Publishing Co., 1898), pp. 48–50.

30 Leith Napier, A. D., *The Menopause and its Disorders* (London: The Scientific Press Ltd, 1897).

31 Ibid., pp. xii, 8, 76–84.

32 Short, R. V., 'Oestrus and menstrual cycles' in Austin, C. R., and Short, R. V., *Reproduction in Mammals. Book 3: Hormonal Control of Reproduction* (Cambridge: CUP, 2nd edn, 1984), ch. 6, pp. 115–52.

33 Moscucci, pp. 18–20, 33–4.

34 Showalter, E. and E., 'Victorian women and menstruation', pp. 38–44, in Vicinus, p. 40. Jules Michelet also accused women of having sabotaged the French Revolution with their religion, superstitions and emotionality.

35 Moscucci, pp. 2–3, 13.

36 Braxton Hicks, J., 'The Croonian Lectures on the difference between the sexes in regard to the aspect and treatment of disease' in *BMJ*, 21 April 1877, 475–6.

37 Vertinsky, p. 93.

38 *The Oxford Companion to Medicine* (1986) says that gynaecology is the study of diseases peculiar to women, i.e. diseases of the ovaries, Fallopian

tubes, uterus (body and cervix), vagina and vulva. The breasts are not usually included except where disease affects them just after childbirth. Today's gynaecologists look at psychology, sociology, environment and relationships (family, social and working) when treating patients.

39 Ibid., pp. 30, 103.

40 Vertinsky, p. 91.

41 Ehrenreich, B., and English, D., *For Her Own Good: 150 Years of the Expert's Advice to Women* (London: Pluto Press, 1979).

42 Walker, p. 172.

43 Wear, A., 'Making sense of health and the environment in early modern England' in Wear, A. (ed.), *Medicine in Society* (Cambridge: CUP, 1992), pp. 119–47; Laqueur, T., and Gallagher, C., *The Making of the Modern Body: Sexuality and Society in the Nineteenth Century* (Berkeley: University of California Press, 1987).

5 Knives and Asylums

1 Porter, R., *The Cambridge Illustrated History of Medicine* (Cambridge: CUP, 1996), pp. 219, 236–7.

2 In another indication of medical attitudes to black slaves the prominent American physician Benjamin Rush suggested that black skin, 'negritude', was itself a disease, akin to leprosy.

3 Harman, C., *Fanny Burney, A Biography* (London: HarperCollins, 2000), pp. 304–7.

4 Dally, A., *Women Under the Knife: A History of Surgery* (London: Hutchinson Radius, 1991), p. 26.

5 Theriot, N. M., 'Women's voices in nineteenth-century medical discourse: A step toward deconstructing science', 12, 15, 24, fn 15, in *Signs*, 19 (1) (Autumn 1993), 1–31.

6 Moscucci, O., *The Science of Women: Gynaecology and Gender in England, 1800–1929* (Cambridge: CUP, 1990), pp. 136–7.

7 Ibid., pp. 136–7, 152.

8 Walton, J., Beeson, B., and Bodley Scott, R. (eds.), *The Oxford Companion to Medicine* (Oxford: OUP, 1986), vol. 1, pp. 236–7.

9 Moscucci, pp. 158, 161–4.

10 Groneman, C., 'Nymphomania: The historical construction of female sexuality' in *Signs: Journal of Women in Culture and Society*, 19 (2) (Winter 1994), 343, 346.

11 Hicks, J. B., 'On the difference between the sexes in regard to the aspect and treatment of disease' in *BMJ* (1877), 1, 413.

12 Medvei, V. C., *A History of Endocrinology* (Lancaster, UK: MTP Press Ltd, 1982), p. 215.

13 Gynaecologists still 'might find it difficult to explain the perception and idiosyncrasies of a woman', see Gurucharri, C. A., 'Culture and medical consultation' in *The Menopause at the Millennium: Proceedings of the 9th International Menopause Society World Congress on the Menopause* (London: Parthenon Publishing, 1999), p. 229.

14 Marañón, G., trans. Stevens, K. S., *The Climacteric (The Critical Age)* (St Louis: C. V. Mosby, 1929), pp. 2, 4, 211.

15 Stewart, M. L., *For Health and Beauty: Physical Culture for Frenchwomen, 1880s–1930s* (Baltimore: The Johns Hopkins University Press, 2001), p. 135.

16 Walton, et al., p. 507.

17 Poovey, M., *Uneven Developments: The Ideological Work of Gender in Mid-Victorian England* (Chicago: University of Chicago Press, 1988), pp. 37–9.

18 Moscucci, pp. 113–14.

19 Wilbush, J., 'Climacteric disorders – historical perspectives' in Studd, J. W. W., and Whitehead, M. I. (eds.), *The Menopause* (Oxford: Blackwell Scientific Publications, 1988), p. 6.

20 *Lancet*, 1 June 1850 and 25 July 1857; Medical Society of London, 1 February 1851.

21 *Lancet*, 27 February 1858; *BMJ*, 23 June 1877.

22 Tilt, E. J., *Handbook of Uterine Therapeutics* (London, 1863).

23 Lawson Tait, R., *Diseases of Women* (London and Edinburgh: Williams and Norgate, 1877), p. 63.

24 Ehrenreich, B., and English, D., *For Her Own Good: 150 Years of the Expert's Advice to Women* (London: Pluto Press, 1979), p. 81.

25 Stopes, M. C., *The Change of Life in Men and Women* (London: Putnam, 1936), p. 206.

26 Micale, M. S., 'On the "disappearance" of hysteria: A study in the clinical deconstruction of a diagnosis' in *Isis*, 84 (3) (September 1993), 496–526, *passim*.

27 Groneman, C., *Nymphomania, a History* (London: Fusion Press, 2001), pp. 7–8.

28 Ashwell, S., *Practical Treatise on the Diseases Peculiar to Women* (London: S. Highley, 1844), pp. 209, 220.

29 Poovey, p. 37.

30 Marañón, p. 204.

31 Barreca, R., *Desire and Imagination: Classic Essays in Sexuality* (London:

Penguin, 1995), pp. 33, 122, 133, 260. Richard von Krafft-Ebing (1840–1902) had a great impact on the works of Adler, Jung and Ellis among others.

32 Ibid., pp. 104–5.

33 Groneman, C., 'Nymphomania: The historical construction of female sexuality' in *Signs: Journal of Women in Culture and Society*, 19 (2) (Winter 1994), 367.

34 Ibid., 338, 343.

35 Shepherd, J., *Lawson Tait: The Rebellious Surgeon* (Lawrence, Kansas: Coronado Press, 1980), p. 52.

36 Barreca, pp. 87–8.

37 Showalter, E., *The Female Malady: Women, Madness and English Culture, 1830–1980* (London: Virago Press, 1987), pp. 75–8.

38 Scull, A., and Favreau, D., 'The cliterodectomy craze' in *Social Research*, 53 (2) (Summer 1986), 243–60.

39 Showalter, p. 78.

40 Groneman, 366.

41 Ibid., 346–7.

42 Ehrenreich and English, p. 104.

43 Moscucci, p. 158. Elizabeth Blackwell opened a dispensary on New York's Lower East Side and, in 1871, established the National Health Society in London to improve the health of the working classes. A purist with a 'Christian physiology' approach, Blackwell believed that there was a connection between physical and moral health. In her book *The Human Element in Sex* (1884), she adamantly argued that medicine could not become an end in itself but needed to understand and incorporate moral law. Mort, F., *Dangerous Sexualities: Medico-moral Politics in England since 1830* (London: Routledge, 2000), p. 86.

44 Ehrenreich and English, p. 57.

45 Moscucci, pp. 37–40.

46 Tyler Smith, W., 'The climacteric disease in women: A cerebral disorder not hitherto described' in *London Journal of Medicine*, 1 (1849), 497, under 'Obstetrics' in the 'Critical Digest of the Journals'.

47 Lawson Tait, p. 148.

48 Ibid., p. 150.

49 Strange, J-M., 'Menstrual fictions: Languages of medicine and menstruation, c. 1850–1930' in *Women's History Review* (2000), 9 (3), 607–28.

50 Theriot, 1–31.

51 Ibid.

52 Scull and Favreau, p. 244.

53 Featherstone, M., and Hepworth, M., 'The history of the male menopause 1848–1936' in *Maturitas* (1985), 7, 249–57.

54 Compton Burnett, J., *The Change of Life in Women and the Ills and Ailings Incident Thereto* (London: The Homeopathic Publishing Co., 1898), pp. 108-10. While homeopathy can help a diseased mind, 'strictly speaking we cannot cure diseases at all. We can, however, cure people whose states and conditions bear man-given names, such as insanity, hyperaesthesia, a cold, rheumatism, or what not. It lies in the nature of things that we should think and talk of diseases as entities, and just as every baby gets a name, so does every disease.'

55 Shepherd, A., 'The female patient experience in two late-nineteenth-century Surrey asylums' in Andrews, J., and Digby, A., *Sex and Seclusion, Class and Custody: Perspectives on Gender and Doctors in the History of British and Irish Psychiatry* (London: Clio Medica, 2004). In France the forty-five- to fifty-year-old woman dominated the lists of female asylum committals who were not classed as 'idiots', see Ripa, Y. (trans.), Catherine du Peloux Menagé, *Women and Madness: The Incarceration of Women in Nineteenth-Century France* (Cambridge: Polity Press, 1990), p. 51.

56 Thompson, D., *Queen Victoria: Gender and Power* (London: Virago, 2001).

57 Ripa, pp. 51–3.

58 Showalter, pp. 55–6, 78, 125. The lives of female inmates were often ones of grinding poverty, which may well have affected their mental health. At Colney Hatch Asylum in 1852, for example, the female attendants were paid £15 a year with board, lodging and laundry, whilst male attendants received £25 with the same benefits.

59 Strange, p. 622.

60 Shepherd, pp. 238–9.

61 According to Freud, 'hysteria' is a form of psychoneurosis in which a repressed emotional conflict finds external expression in sensory and motor dysfunction such as loss of sensation over parts of the body, temporary blindness, paralysis of limbs, loss or impairment of speech and hearing, or even convulsions. It is an anxiety neurosis which is accompanied by the 'most distinct diminution of the sexual libido or the psychic desire'. Selective memory loss for personal events may also occur, including loss of personal identity or an hysterical 'fugue'. Hysterics occasionally display an incongruous lack of concern for their disability ('la belle indifference'). See Walton, et al.; Brill, A. (trans.), *Freud's Sel. Papers on Hysteria* (London: Allen & Unwin, 1948), vi, p. 147. Maines, R. P.,

The Technology of Orgasm: 'Hysteria', the Vibrator, and Women's Sexual Satisfaction (Baltimore: The Johns Hopkins University Press, 1999), p. 45.

62 Micale, pp. 496–7, 501.

63 Marañón, pp. 227, 229.

64 Ibid., pp. 496–7, 501, 523, 525.

65 Theriot, pp. 110–11, 125.

6 Sex, Science and Sensibility

1 Ladimer, B., *Colette, Beauvoir, and Duras: Age and Women Writers* (Gainesville: University Press of Florida, 1999), p. 202.

2 Haller, J. S., and Haller, R. M., *The Physician and Sexuality in Victorian America* (Champaign: University of Illinois Press, 1974), p. 46.

3 Napheys, G., *The Physical Life of Women* (London, 1893).

4 Groneman, C., 'Nymphomania: The historical construction of female sexuality' in *Signs: Journal of Women in Culture and Society*, 19 (2), 339.

5 Bullough, V., and Voght, M., 'Women, menstruation and nineteenth-century medicine', 67 in *Bulletin of the History of Medicine*, 47 (1) (Spring 1973), 66–82.

6 Oudshoorn, N., *Beyond the Natural Body: An Archeology of Sex Hormones* (London: Routledge, 1994), pp. 2, 16.

7 Bullough and Voght, pp. 78–9.

8 Haller and Haller, pp. 134–5.

9 Medvei, V. C., *A History of Endocrinology* (Lancaster, UK: MTP Press Ltd, 1982), p. 364.

10 Compton Burnett, J., *The Change of Life in Women and the Ills and Ailings Incident Thereto* (London: The Homeopathic Publishing Co., 1898), pp. 86–8.

11 Fausto-Sterling, A., *Sexing the Body: Gender Politics and the Construction of Sexuality* (New York: Basic Books, 2000), p. 170.

12 Medvei, p. 189.

13 Oudshoorn, p. 16.

14 Medvei, pp. 373, 375, 396, 501.

15 *The Oxford Companion to Medicine*, vol. 1, pp. 336–8.

16 Medvei, p. 4.

17 Sengoopta, C., 'Secrets of eternal youth' in *History Today*, 56 (August 2006), 50–6.

18 Stewart, M. L., *For Health and Beauty: Physical Culture for Frenchwomen, 1880s–1930s* (Baltimore: The Johns Hopkins University Press, 2001), pp. 139–41.

19 Oudshoorn, p. 60.

20 Medvei, pp. 401–3. Zondek described the role of ovarian hormones at menopause as an excessive secretion of oestrin which could last for months, followed by a decline characterized by vasomotor instability, and then an increase of secretion of pituitary gonadotrophic hormone, which could remain permanently in the urine. These stages, he considered, merged imperceptibly with each other.

21 Oudshoorn, pp. 42–3.

22 Ibid., pp. 107–8.

23 Bell, S. E., 'Changing ideas: The medicalization of menopause' in *Social Science & Medicine* (1987), 24 (6), 535–42.

24 Parker, E., *The Seven Ages of Woman* (Baltimore: The Johns Hopkins Press, 1960).

25 Gold, J., *The Psychiatric Implications of Menstruation* (Washington, DC: American Psychiatric Press Inc., 1986), p. 98.

26 Budoff, P. W., 'Cyclic estrogen-progesterone therapy' in Walsh, M. R., *The Psychology of Women* (New Haven: Yale University Press, 1987), pp. 150–6.

27 Rogers, J., *Endocrine and Metabolic Aspects of Gynaecology* (Philadelphia: Saunders, 1963), pp. 118–19, 121, 130.

28 Sarah Wildman in *TNR* (*The New Republic*) Online, July 2002.

29 Studd, J. W. W., and Whitehead, M. I. (eds.), *The Menopause* (Oxford: Blackwell Scientific Publications, 1988), p. viii.

30 Seaman, B., and Seaman, G., *Women and the Crisis in Sex Hormones. An Investigation of the Dangerous Uses of Hormones from Birth Control to Menopause, and the Safe Alternatives* (Sussex: The Harvester Press Ltd, 1978).

31 Haller and Haller, pp. 47, 84.

7 A Question of 'Male Menopause'

1 'Viropause' – *Food and Fitness: A Dictionary of Diet and Exercise*, Michael Kent, Oxford University Press, 1997. *Oxford Reference Online* – http://www.oxford-reference.com/views/ENTRY.html?subview=Main&entry=t38.e1810; Zichella, L., Whitehead, M. I., and van Keep, P. A. (eds.), *The Climacteric and Beyond* (Proceedings of the 5th International Congress on the Menopause 1987 . . . under the auspices of the International Menopause Society), p. 85.

2 McLaren, A., *Impotence: A Cultural History* (Chicago: The University of Chicago Press, 2007), p. 51.

3 Corfe, G., *Man and His Many Changes or, Seven Times Seven* (London: Houlston and Wright, 1849), p. 73.

4 Acton, William, *The Functions and Disorders of the Reproductive Organs* (London, 1857). More recently, medicine has not been above using biblical

anecdote in its support – Joel Wilbush has quoted Kings 1, 1: 1–4: 'The elderly male is less vigorous in his sex life, even in the presence of an attractive partner, a fact that has been documented since biblical time.' And he has enlisted the classics, too, using Cicero's truism 'Sic se res habet; ut enim non omne vinum, sic non omnis natura vetustate coacescit', from *De Senectute* ('An Essay on Old Age'). But this statement is about character, not age, about the tendency of old men to be anxious, jittery, grumpy, avaricious and nasty.

5 Medvei, V. C., *A History of Endocrinology* (Lancaster, UK: MTP Press Ltd, 1982), pp. 289–90.

6 Hormones circulate via a 'canal system' in the body. Circulation of the blood was first described by William Harvey at the beginning of the seventeenth century but it was another 250 years before it was understood that all organs communicate with each other via this system. This chemical communication is the sole function of particular organs, most especially the glands with their complicated regulatory endocrine mechanism. Medvei, p. 3, suggests this is the natural child of the humoural doctrine.

7 Lock, S., '"O that I were young again": Yeats and the Steinach operation' in *BMJ*, 287 (24–31 December 1983), 1964–7. Sengoopta, C., 'Secrets of Eternal Youth' in *History Today*, 56 (August 2006), 54. Steinach mentioned some 2000 vasectomies performed by 1940 in Vienna, New York, London, St Petersburg, Copenhagen, Chile, Cuba and India. Steinach advocated his surgical procedures as a way of retaining vigour and vitality, and in this he harked back to traditionally held ideas of the weakening effects of spilling semen.

8 Marañón, G., trans. Stevens, K., *The Climacteric (The Critical Age)* (St Louis: C. V. Mosby, 1929), pp. 349–76.

9 Featherstone, M., and Hepworth, M., 'The history of the menopause 1848–1936' in *Maturitas* (1985), 7, 251–2.

10 Hall, R. (ed.), *Dear Doctor Stopes: Sex in the 1920s* (London: Andre Deutsch, 1978).

11 Stopes, M. C., *Change of Life in Men and Women* (London: Putnam, 1936), pp. 47–8, 58–9, 64.

12 Ibid., pp. 91, 113, 244.

13 Walton, J., Beeson, B., and Bodley Scott, R. (eds.), *The Oxford Companion to Medicine* (Oxford: OUP, 1986), vol. 1, pp. 337–8.

14 Oudshoorn, N., *Beyond the Natural Body: An Archeology of Sex Hormones* (London: Routledge, 1944), p. 104.

15 Heller, C. G., and Myers, G. B., 'The male climacteric, its symptomatology, diagnosis and treatment' in *JAMA* (1944), 126, 472–7.

16 McLaren, A., *Impotence: A Cultural History* (Chicago: The University of Chicago Press, 2007), pp. 210, 222.

17 Ibid., pp. 235–57.

18 Ibid.

19 Gould, D. C., Petty, R., and Jacobs, H. S., 'The male menopause – does it exist?' in *BMJ* (2000), 320, 858–61.

20 Drazin, C. (ed.), *John Fowles, The Journals, Volume 2* (London: Vintage, 2007), pp. 383, 398.

21 In 2007 Pfizer launched a 'new diagnostic tool', the Erectile Hardness Score (EHS), to measure erectile hardness on a scale of 1 to 4: Grade 1 – Penis is larger but not hard; Grade 2 – Penis is hard, but not hard enough for penetration; Grade 3 – Penis is hard enough for penetration but not completely hard; and Grade 4 – Penis is completely hard and fully rigid. In validation, the EHS was shown to correlate strongly with ED status as defined by the International Index of Erectile Function: Grade 1 – Severe ED; Grade 2 – Moderate ED; Grade 3 – Mild ED; and Grade 4 – No ED. The launch was reported in an article by Mulhall, J., et al., 'Erectile dysfunction: Monitoring response to treatment in clinical practice – recommendations of an international study panel' in *Journal of Sexual Medicine* (2007), 4, 448–64.

22 See, for example, a review of the *BMJ* article by Dr Robert W. Griffith at www.healthandage.com

23 www.studd.co.uk

24 According to Cancer Research UK prostate cancer is the most common cancer in men, accounting for nearly a quarter (23 per cent) of all new male cancer diagnoses. Increased detection (through PSA, prostate specific antigen tests) of the illness has led to the huge rise in incidence over the last twenty years. The lifetime risk of being diagnosed with this cancer is 1 in 14 for men in the UK and is strongly related to age; very few men under fifty are at risk whilst more than 60 per cent of cases occur in men over seventy years old. But only 1 in 25 men (4 per cent) will die from this disease, meaning that men are more likely to die with it than from it. The extremely high rate of incidence in the USA (125 per 100,000) is more than twice the reported rate in the UK (52 per 100,000) but is likely to be due to the high rates of PSA testing in America. Black American men have higher rates than white American men, and a study of rates of prostate cancer mortality in Jewish

American men found they were significantly lower than for non-Jewish white Americans. See www.info.cancerresearchuk.org/cancerstats/types/prostate/incidence

8   Finding a Voice

1   Stopes, M. C., *Change of Life in Men and Women* (London: Putnam, 1936), p. 269.

2   *Oxford Dictionary of National Biography*.

3   Dulberg, Joseph, *Sterile Marriage: The Various Causes which Produce Childlessness . . . the Menopause (Change of Life)* (London: T. Werner Laurie Ltd, 1920), pp. 145–70.

4   Marañón, G., trans. Stevens, K., *The Climacteric (The Critical Age)*, (St Louis: C. V. Mosby, 1929), p. 198.

5   Ibid., pp. 125–6, 385

6   Ibid., pp. 198–202.

7   Ibid., pp. 210–11.

8   Ibid., pp. 202–3.

9   Bell, A. O. (ed.), introduction by Quentin Bell, *The Diary of Virginia Woolf* (London: Hogarth Press, 1977–84), vol. 5, 1936–41.

10 Woolf, V. (1882–1941), *Mrs Dalloway*, introduction by Elaine Showalter (London: Penguin, 2000).

11 Showalter remarks that the male characters approach ageing very differently, having 'the chance to renew their lives through action' rather than having to 'live their lives vicariously through their daughters' as women often did.

12 Kent, S. K., 'Gender reconstruction after the First World War' in *British Feminism in the Twentieth Century*, ed. Smith, H. L. (Aldershot: Edward Elgar Publishing Ltd, 1990), p. 71.

13 Davidson, C. N., and Wagner-Martin, L., 'Menopause' in *The Oxford Companion to Women's Writing in the United States* (Oxford: OUP, 1995).

14 Stopes, pp. 7–8.

15 Ibid., p. 130.

16 'Medica', *Change of Life: Facts and Fallacies of Middle Age* (London: Delisle, 1948), pp. 5–6, 28.

17 Ibid., p. 7.

18 Stopes, p. 244.

19 Maines, R. P., *The Technology of Orgasm: 'Hysteria', the Vibrator, and Women's Sexual Satisfaction* (Baltimore: The Johns Hopkins University Press, 1999), pp. 86–7, 95.

20 Stopes, p. 135.

21 Ibid., pp. 3–4.

22 Bullough, V. L., 'The development of sexology in the USA' in Porter, R., and Teich, M. (eds.), *Sexual Knowledge, Sexual Science: A History of Attitudes to Sexuality* (Cambridge: CUP, 1994), pp. 303–23.

23 Stopes, p. 26.

24 From her paper 'The sexual variety and variability among women and their bearing upon social reconstruction', given to the British Society for (the Study of) Sex Psychology on 14 October 1915.

25 Stopes, p. 180.

26 Ibid., p. 196.

27 Deutsch, H., *The Psychology of Women* (London: Research Books Ltd, 1946).

28 Parker, E., *The Seven Ages of Women* (Baltimore: The Johns Hopkins Press, 1960).

29 'Medica', p. 3.

30 'Menopause, mortgages and Mrs Thatcher' by Jenni Murray, celebrating sixty years of *Woman's Hour* in September 2006, in the *Guardian*.

31 Carr, D. E., *The Sexes* (London: Heinemann, 1971), p. 114.

32 Houck, J. A., '"What do these women want?": Feminist responses to *Feminine Forever*, 1963–1980' in *Bulletin of the History of Medicine*, 77 (1) (Spring 2003), 103–32.

33 Dillaway, H. E., 'When does menopause occur, and how long does it last? Wrestling with age- and time-based conceptualizations of reproductive aging' in *NWSA Journal* (Spring 2006), 18 (1), 31–61.

34 Houck, p. 110.

35 Ibid.

36 Ibid., pp. 110–12.

37 Ibid.

38 Gold, J., *The Psychiatric Implications of Menstruation* (Washington, DC: American Psychiatric Press Inc., 1986), p. 98.

39 Zichella, L., Whitehead, M. I., and van Keep, P. A. (eds.), *The Climacteric and Beyond* (Proceedings of the 5th International Congress on the Menopause 1987 . . . under the auspices of the International Menopause Society), pp. 155, 166.

9 Fear or Freedom

1 Popper, K., 'The logic and evolution of a scientific theory' in *All Life is Problem Solving* (London: Routledge, 1999), pp. 3–22, 110.

2 Douglas, M., *Purity and Danger: An Analysis of Concepts of Pollution and Taboo* (London: Routledge, 2003, 1st pub. 1966).

3 MacPherson, K., 'Going to the source: Women reclaim menopause' in *Feminist Studies* (Summer 1995), 21 (2), 347.

4 www.jewishjournal.com Rabbi Debra Orenstein has said that Jewish tradition has been silent about menopause 'and the losses and stresses that [this] . . . represents', including 'getting older, on loss of fertility, on mortality and femininity. Judaism has a lot to teach about these themes'. Using Jewish sources and existing traditions, women have begun to create rituals that recognize menopause ranging from a simple blessing to an elaborate seder. Many draw on Pesach metaphors and mikvah to mark the moving from one stage of life to another. Mikvah represents the womb of the Jewish people, so when one comes to the mikvah it is a rebirth. It is not a question of loss but of gain. 'Making ritual available takes away any aspect of shame', and these rituals 'provide a communal way to address' such major life transitions. If a woman has faithfully observed the mikvah all her adult life it may be that she will experience a heightened sense of loss at menopause.

5 Chirawatkul, S., and Manderson, L., 'Perceptions of menopause in northeast Thailand: Contested meaning and practice' in *Social Science & Medicine* (1994), 39 (11), 1545–54.

6 Conrad, P., *The Medicalization of Society* (Baltimore: The Johns Hopkins University Press, 2007), pp. 121–2.

7 Magliano, D. J., et al., 'Hormone therapy and cardiovascular disease: A systematic review and meta-analysis' in *British Journal of Obstetrics and Gynaecology*, 113 (January 2006), 5.

8 Obesity increases the risk of breast cancer – but only after the menopause. A large European study called Epic found post-menopausal women who were obese had a 31 per cent higher risk of breast cancer than women with a healthy weight. Reducing obesity could save 1800 cases of breast cancer a year.

9 Bell, S. E. 'Changing ideas: The medicalization of menopause' in *Social Science & Medicine* (1987), 24 (6), 535–42.

10 Press release from 2007, www.info.cancerresearchuk.org Professor Valerie Beral, director of Cancer Research UK's epidemiology unit at the University of Oxford, and her colleagues published the results of their study in the *Lancet* in April 2007. The risks of breast cancer are the highest and, in total, ovarian, endometrial and breast cancer account for 39 per cent of all cancers registered in women in the UK. The total incidence of these three cancers in the study population is 63 per cent higher in current users of HRT than in those who have never used the

drugs. The study concluded that HRT leads to a material increase in these common cancers, though when women stop taking the drugs their risk returns to normal.

11   BBC Radio 4, *Woman's Hour*, 9 April 2007.

12   Roberts, P. J., 'The menopause and hormone replacement therapy: Views of women in general practice receiving hormone replacement therapy' in *British Journal of General Practice*, 41 (351) (October 1991), 421–4.

13   Ibid.

14   Black cohosh, one of the most popular herbal remedies, is a plant related to the buttercup and has tall spikes of brilliant white flowers and a gnarled, resin-scented root. It grows wild in the eastern United States – the fact that Native Americans have used it as a folk remedy for centuries is a selling point to those who mistrust science. The Cherokee relied on alcoholic spirits of black cohosh root to treat rheumatism and ground the root into teas to treat consumption and fatigue and the Algonquins used it for kidney trouble – which tallies with Chinese medicine in that menopausal symptoms are related to kidney deficiency. In 1849 the American Medical Association thought it useful for 'the debility of females attendant upon uterine disorder' and 150 years later, following the cancer scares of HRT, sales in America topped $34 million, three times the sales figure of the year before. The leading black cohosh brand, 'RemiFemin', has been available since 1955 and the pharmaceutical giant GlaxoSmithKline has acquired the rights to market it as a dietary supplement in America. Black cohosh contains phytoestrogen, a plant substance that has effects similar to those of oestrogens, but little is known about long-term safety and toxicity. The Japanese, whose diet is high in phytoestrogens (also found in soybeans, chickpeas, red clover and probably other legumes), appear to have lower rates of menopausal vasomotor symptoms, cardio-vascular disease, osteoporosis, and breast, colon, endometrial and ovarian cancers. Dr Wulf Utian, director of the North American Menopause Society, argues that, despite the 'media hype', rigorous studies show little difference between black cohosh and placebos. The jury is, unsurprisingly, still out.

15   In Chinese medicine, increasingly popular as an alternative to Western medicine, the menopause is one of the 'Gateways of Change' (others being birth and early development, puberty, onset of sexual activity, childbirth and post-natal). It is seen as a time for positive development if managed well, but is also regarded as a vulnerable time, when illness

could arise. Blood is a valuable resource and after a lifetime of menstruation a woman's reserves are thought to become depleted – hence signs and symptoms of heat, dryness, restlessness, rising energy, lack of nourishment to hair, nails, skin, brain, and the decrease or absence of menstruation. The transition is supported by a regime to strengthen the spleen which supports blood, via herbs, diet, exercise, stillness, rest and fluids (water), and by reducing heat-producing activities and foods (stress, overwork, hot, spicy foods, alcohol, coffee).

16 www.baaps.org.uk This report was published in February 2008 by BAAPS, based at the Royal College of Surgeons, a 'not-for-profit organisation established for the advancement of education and practice of Aesthetic Plastic Surgery for public benefit'.

17 Stewart, M. L., *For Health and Beauty: Physical Culture for Frenchwomen, 1880s–1930s* (Baltimore: The Johns Hopkins University Press, 2001), pp. 143–4.

18 *Observer*, 29 October 2006, p. 42. The article, by Joanna Walters, reports on the publication of *Beauty Junkies* by Alex Kuczynski, a columnist for the Style section of the *New York Times*.

19 Cherry, K., Jamhour, N., and Mincey, P. B., review of Gullette, M., *Aged by Culture* in *Biography*, 27 (3) (Summer 2004), 631–4.

20 Willson, S., 'Perspectives, theatre in brief' in the *Lancet* (2007), 369, 1782.

BIBLIOGRAPHY

Primary Sources

Anderson, J., *Medical Remarks on Natural, Spontaneous and Artificial Evacuation* (London: printed for the author and sold by J. Murray and by J. Donaldson, Edinburgh, 1787)

Ashwell, S., *Practical Treatise on the Diseases Peculiar to Women* (London: S. Highley, 1844)

Astruc, J., *A Treatise on all the Diseases Incident to Women*, translated from a manuscript copy of the author's lectures read at Paris, 1740, by J. R-n. (London: printed for T. Cooper at the Globe, 1743)

Chadwick, M., *Woman's Periodicity* (London: Douglas, 1933)

Cogan, T., *Haven of Health* (London: printed by Henrie Midleton, for William Norton, 1584)

Compton Burnett, J., *The Change of Life in Women and the Ills and Ailings Incident Thereto* (London: The Homeopathic Publishing Co., 1898)

Corfe, G., *Man and His Many Changes or, Seven Times Seven* (London: Houlston and Wright, 1849)

Crooke, H, *Mikrokosmographia* (London: printed by T. and R. Coates, 1631)

Deutsch, H., *The Psychology of Women* (London: Research Books Ltd, 1946)

Dulberg, J., *Sterile Marriages; the various causes which produce childlessness . . . the menopause (change of life)* (London: T. Werner Laurie Ltd, 1920)

Fontaine, N., *The Womans Doctour or, an exact and distinct Explanation of all such Diseases as peculiar to that Sex. With Choice and Experimentall Remedies against the same. Being Safe in the Composition, Pleasant in the Use, Effectuall in the Operation, Cheap in the Price* (London, 1652)

Freind, J., *Emmenologia* (London: Thomas Bennet, 1703)

Kinsey, A. C., *Sexual Behavior in the Human Female* (Philadelphia: Saunders, 1953)

Lawson Tait, R., *Diseases of Women* (London and Edinburgh: William and Norgate, 1877)

Leake, J., *Medical Instructions Towards the Prevention and Cure of Chronic or Slow Diseases Peculiar to Women: Especially those proceeding from over-delicacy of habit called Nervous or Hysterical; from Female Obstructions, Weakness and inward Decay; a diseased state of the Womb, or critical Change of Constitution at particular Periods of Life, in which, their Nature is explained, and their Treatment by Regimen, and simple Medicines . . .* (London: printed for R. Baldwin, 1777)

Leith Napier, A. D., *The Menopause and its Disorders* (London: The Scientific Press Ltd, 1897)

Levinus Lemnius, *The secret miracles of nature: in four books: learnedly and moderately treating of generation, and the parts thereof, the soul, and its immortality, of plants and living creatures, of diseases, their symptoms and cures, and many other rarities . . . : whereunto is added one book containing philosophical and prudential rules how man shall become excellent in all conditions, whether high or low, and lead his life with health of body and mind / written by that famous physitian, Levinus Lemnius.* (London: printed by Jo Streter, 1658)

Manning, H., *A Treatise of Female Diseases* (London: printed for R. Baldwin, 1771)

Marañón, G., trans. Stevens, K. S., *The Climacteric (The Critical Age)* (St Louis: C. V. Mosby, 1929)

'Medica', *Change of Life: Facts and Fallacies of Middle Age* (London: Delisle, 1948)

Medico-Chirurgical Transactions, 77 (1894)

Napheys, G., *The Physical Life of Women* (London, 1893)

Novak, E., *The Woman Asks the Doctor* (London, 1936)

Parker, E., *The Seven Ages of Woman* (Baltimore: The Johns Hopkins Press, 1960)

Robertson, J., *Essays and Notes on the Physiology and Diseases of Women, and on Practical Midwifery* (London, 1851)

Rogers, J., *Endocrine and Metabolic Aspects of Gynaecology* (Philadelphia and London: Saunders, 1963)

Sadler, J., *The Sicke Womans Private Looking-Glasse wherein Methodically are handled all uterine affects, or diseases arising from the Wombe; enabling Women to informe the Physician about the cause of their griefe* (London: printed by Anne Griffin for Philemon Stephens and Christopher Meridith, 1636)

Saville, G., *The Lady's New Year's Gift, Or, Advice to a Daughter* (1707)

Tilt, E, J., *The Change of Life in Health and Disease. A Practical Treatise on the Nervous and Other Affections Incidental to Women at the Decline of Life* (London: John Churchill, 1857)

——*Handbook of Uterine Therapeutics* (London, 1863)

Transactions of the Obstetrical Society of London, 36 (1894)

Tyler-Smith, W., 'The Climacteric Disease of Women' in *London Journal of Medicine*, I (1848), 601

Walker, A., *Beauty: Illustrated Chiefly by an Analysis and Classification of Beauty in Woman* (London: E. Wilson, 1836)

Woolley, H., *The Gentlewomans Companion or, a Guide to the Female Sex: containing Directions of Behaviour, in all Places, Companies, Relations, and Conditions, from their Childhood down to Old Age* (London: printed by A. Maxwell for Edward Thomas . . . , 1675)

Secondary Sources

Abbott, E., *A History of Celibacy* (Cambridge: Butterworth Press, 2001)

Anderson, O., *Suicide in Victorian and Edwardian England* (Oxford, Clarendon Press, 1987)

Andrews, J., and Digby, A., *Sex and Seclusion, Class and Custody: Perspectives on Gender and Doctors in the History of British and Irish Psychiatry* (London: Clio Medica, 2004)

Apter, T., *Secret Paths: Women in the New Midlife* (London: W.W. Norton & Company, 1995)

Austin, C. R., and Short, R. V., *Reproduction in Mammals. Book 3: Hormonal Control of Reproduction* (Cambridge: CUP, 2nd edn, 1984)

Barreca, R., *Desire and Imagination: Classic Essays in Sexuality* (London: Penguin, 1995)

Bell, A. O., (ed.), introduced by Quentin Bell, *The Diary of Virginia Woolf* (London: Hogarth Press, 1977–84)

Bell, S. G., and Offen, K. M. (eds.), *Women, the Family, and Freedom: The Debate in Documents, vol. 1: 1750–1880* (Stanford: Stanford University Press, 1983)

Berger, G. E., *Menopause and Culture* (London: Pluto, 1999)

Burns, J. H. (ed.), *The Cambridge History of Medieval Political Thought c. 350–c. 1450* (Cambridge: CUP, 1991)

Cameron, A., and Kuhrt, A. (eds.), *Images of Women in Antiquity* (London: Routledge, 1991)

Carr, D. E., *The Sexes* (London: Heinemann, 1971)

Cohn, N., *The Pursuit of the Millenium: Revolutionary Millenarians and Mystical Anarchists of the Middle Ages* (London: Maurice Temple Smith Ltd, 1970)

Coney, S., *The Menopause Industry: A Guide to Medicine's 'Discovery' of the Mid-life Woman* (London: Women's Press, 1995)

Conrad, P., *The Medicalization of Society: On the Transformation of Human Conditions into Treatable Disorders* (Baltimore: The Johns Hopkins University Press, 2007)

Dally, A., *Women Under the Knife: A History of Surgery* (London: Hutchinson Radius, 1991)

Dean-Jones, L., *Women's Bodies in Classical Greek Science* (Oxford: OUP, 1994)

Drazin, C. (ed.), *John Fowles, The Journals, Volume 2* (London: Vintage, 2007)

Eadie, M. J., and Bladin, P. F., *A Disease Once Sacred: A History of the Medical Understanding of Epilepsy* (Eastleigh: John Libbey & Co. Ltd, 2001)

Ehrenreich, B., and English, D., *Complaints and Disorders: The Sexual Politics of Sickness* (London: Writers and Readers Publishing Cooperative, 1976)

——*For Her Own Good: 150 Years of the Expert's Advice to Women* (London: Pluto Press, 1979)

Fausto-Sterling, A., *Sexing the Body: Gender Politics and the Construction of Sexuality* (New York: Basic Books, 2000)

Flemming, R., *Medicine and the Making of Roman Women: Gender, Nature, and Authority from Celsus to Galen* (Oxford: OUP, 2000)

Foxcroft, L., *The Making of Addiction: The Use and Abuse of Opium in Nineteenth-Century Britain* (Aldershot: Ashgate Publishing Ltd, 2007)

Gannon, L. R., *Women and Aging: Transcending the Myths* (London: Routledge, 1999)

Gatrell, V. A. C., *City of Laughter: Sex and Satire in Eighteenth-Century London* (London: Atlantic Books, 2006)

Godbeer, R., *The Devil's Dominion: Magic and Religion in Early New England* (Cambridge: CUP, 1992)

Gold, J. M., *The Psychiatric Implications of Menstruation* (Washington, DC: American Psychiatric Press Inc., 1986)

Goodman, A., *Margery Kempe and Her World* (London: Pearson Education Ltd, 2002)

Green, Monica, ed., *Women's Health Care in the Medieval West* (Aldershot: Ashgate Publishing Ltd, 2000)

——(ed., trans.), *The Trotula: A Medieval Compendium of Women's Medicine* (Philadelphia: University of Pennsylvania Press, 2001)

Greer, G., *The Change: Women, Ageing and the Menopause* (London: Hamish Hamilton, 1991)

Groneman, C., *Nymphomania, a History* (London: Fusion Press, 2001)

Gullette, M. M., *Aged by Culture* (Chicago: University of Chicago Press, 2004)

Hall, R. (ed.), *Dear Doctor Stopes: Sex in the 1920s* (London, Andre Deutsch, 1978)

Haller, J. S., and Haller, R. M., *The Physician and Sexuality in Victorian America* (Champaign: University of Illinois Press, 1974)

Hankinson, R. J. (ed.), *Galen* (Cambridge: CUP, 2008)

Harman, C., *Fanny Burney, A Biography* (London: HarperCollins, 2000)

Heinemann, E., *Witches: A Psychoanalytic Exploration of the Killing of Women*, trans. D. Kiraly (London: Free Association Books, 2000)

Houck, J. A., *Hot and Bothered: Women, Medicine, and Menopause in the United States* (Cambridge, Mass.: Harvard University Press, 2006)

Hufton, O., *The Prospect Before Her: A History of Women in Western Europe, Volume 1, 1500–1800* (London: HarperCollins, 1995)

Kirkwood, T., *Time of Our Lives: The Science of Human Ageing* (London: Weidenfield and Nicolson, 1999)

Komesaroff, P. A., Rothfield, P., and Daly, J. (eds.), *Reinterpreting Menopause: Cultural and Philosophical Issues* (London: Routledge, 1997)

Ladimer, B., *Colette, Beauvoir, and Duras: Age and Women Writers* (Gainesville: University Press of Florida, 1999)

Laqueur, T., and Gallagher, C., *The Making of the Modern Body: Sexuality and Society in the Nineteenth Century* (Berkeley: University of California Press, 1987)

Levack, B. P., *Witch-hunt in Early Modern Europe* (London: Longman, 1995)

Levy, M., *The Moons of Paradise: Some Reflections on the Appearance of the Female Breast in Art* (London: A. Barker, 1962)

Maines, R. P., *The Technology of Orgasm: 'Hysteria', the Vibrator, and Women's Sexual Satisfaction* (Baltimore: The Johns Hopkins University Press, 1999)

Mastroianni, L., and Paulsen, C. A. (eds.), *Aging, Reproduction, and the Climacteric* (New York: Plenum Press, 1986)

McLaren, A., *Impotence: A Cultural History* (Chicago: The University of Chicago Press, 2007)

Medvei, V. C., *A History of Endocrinology* (Lancaster, UK: MTP Press Ltd, 1982)

Mort, F., *Dangerous Sexualities: Medico-moral Politics in England since 1830* (Routledge, 2000)

Moscucci, O. *The Science of Women: Gynaecology and Gender in England, 1800–1929* (Cambridge: CUP, 1990)

Murray, J., *Is it Me or is it Hot in Here? A Modern Woman's Guide to Menopause* (London: Vermilion, 2001)

Nutton, V., *Ancient Medicine* (London: Routledge, 2004)

Orr, L., *Jules Michelet: Nature, History, and Language* (Ithaca: Cornell University Press, 1976)

Oudshoorn, N., *Beyond the Natural Body: An Archeology of Sex Hormones* (London: Routledge, 1994)

Oxford Dictionary of National Biography (Oxford: OUP, 2004–6)

Parry, V., *The Truth About Hormones* (London: Atlantic Books, 2005)

Pennell, S., *Women in Medicine: Remedy Books, 1533–1865* (Wellcome Library, London, Primary Source Microfilm)

Poovey, M , *Uneven Developments: The Ideological Work of Gender in Mid-Victorian England* (Chicago: University of Chicago Press, 1988)

Popper, K., *All Life is Problem Solving* (London: Routledge, 1999)

Porter, R., *Mind-Forg'd Manacles: A History of Madness in England from the Restoration to the Regency* (London: Penguin Books, 1990)

——, *The Cambridge Illustrated History of Medicine* (Cambridge: CUP, 1996)

Porter, R., and Bynum, W. F. (eds.), *Medical Fringe and Medical Orthodoxy* (London: Routledge, 1987)

Porter, R., and Teich, M. (eds.), *Sexual Knowledge, Sexual Science: A History of Attitudes to Sexuality* (Cambridge: CUP, 1994)

Ripa, Y. (trans.), Catherine du Peloux Menagé, *Women and Madness: The Incarceration of Women in Nineteenth-century France* (Cambridge: Polity Press, 1990)

Rowland, B., *Medieval Woman's Guide to Health: The First English Gynecological Handbook* (London: Crook Helm, 1981)

Shepherd, J., *Lawson Tait: The Rebellious Surgeon* (Coronado Press, 1980)

Shorter, E., *A History of Women's Bodies* (London: Allen Lane, 1983)

Showalter, E., *The Female Malady: Women, Madness and English Culture, 1830–1980* (London: Virago Press, 1987)

Skinner, H. A., *The Origin of Medical Terms* (Baltimore: Williams & Wilkins, 1970)

Smith, H. (ed.), *British Feminism in the Twentieth Century* (Aldershot: Elgar, 1990)

Smith-Rosenberg, C., *Disorderly Conduct: Visions of Gender in Victorian America* (Oxford: OUP, 1986)

St Clair, W., and Maassen, I. (eds.), *Conduct Literature for Women 1500–1640* (London: Pickering & Chatto, c. 2000)

Steinem, G., *Revolution from Within: A Book of Self-esteem* (London: Bloomsbury, 1992)

Stewart, M. L., *For Health and Beauty: Physical Culture for Frenchwomen, 1880s–1930s* (Baltimore: The Johns Hopkins University Press, 2001)

Stopes, M. C., *Change of Life in Men and Women* (London: Putnam, 1936)

Studd, J. W. W., and Whitehead, M. I. (eds.), *The Menopause* (Oxford: Blackwell Scientific Publications, 1988)

Szasz, Thomas, *The Myth of Mental Illness: Foundations of a Theory of Personal Conduct* (London: Secker & Warburg, 1962)

te Velde, E. R,. Pearson, P. L., and Broekmans, F. J. (eds.), *Female Reproductive Aging. Studies in Profertility Series Vol. 9. The Proceedings of the 10th Reinier de Graaf Symposium, Zeist, The Netherlands, 9–11 September 1999* (London: Parthenon Publishing Group, 2000)

Thompson, D., *Queen Victoria: Gender and Power* (London, Virago, 2001)

Trevor-Roper, H. R., *The European Witch-Craze of the Sixteenth and Seventeenth Century* (London: Penguin Books, 1990)

Trumbach, R. (ed.), *Marriage, Sex and the Family in England, 1660–1800* (New York: Garland Publishing Inc., 1986)

Vertinsky, P., *The Eternally Wounded Woman: Women, Doctors and Exercise in the Late Nineteenth Century* (Manchester: Manchester University Press, 1990)

Vicinus, M., (ed.), *Suffer and Be Still: Women in the Victorian Age* (Bloomington: Indiana University Press, 1972)

Walkowitz, J. R., *Prostitution and Victorian Society: Women, Class, and the State* (Cambridge: CUP, 1980)

Walsh, M. R., *The Psychology of Women* (New Haven: Yale University Press, 1987)

Walton, J., Beeson, P. B., and Bodley Scott R. (eds.), *The Oxford Companion to Medicine* (Oxford: OUP, 1986), vols. 1 and 2

Wasserfall, R. (ed.), *Women and Water: Menstruation in Jewish Life and Law* (Hanover, New Hampshire: University Press of New England, 1999)

Weeks, Jeffrey, *Sex, Politics and Society* (London: Longman Publishing Group, 1989)

Weisner, M., *Women and Gender in Early Modern Europe* Cambridge: CUP, 2000)

Wilson, R. A., *Feminine Forever* (London: WH Allen, 1966)

Woolf, V., *Mrs Dalloway*, with an introduction by Elaine Showalter (London: Penguin, 2000)

Zichella, L., Whitehead, M. I., and van Keep, P. A. (eds.), *The Climacteric and Beyond* (Proceedings of the 5th International Congress on the Menopause 1987 . . . under the auspices of the International Menopause Society)

Articles

Althof, S. E., Dean, J., Derogatis, L. R., Rosen, R. C., and Sisson, M., 'Current perspectives on the clinical assessment and diagnosis of female sexual dysfunction and clinical studies of potential therapies: A statement of concern' in *The Journal of Sexual Medicine*, 2 (September 2005), 146

Amundsen, D. W., and Diers, C. J., 'The age of menopause in medieval Europe' in *Human Biology* (December 1973), 45 (4), 605–612

Avis, N., Stellato, R., Crawford, S., Bromberger, J., Ganz, P., Cain, V., and Kagaw-Singer, M., 'Is there a menopausal syndrome? Menopausal status and symptoms across racial/ethnic groups' in *Social Science & Medicine* (2001), 52, 345–56.

Basson, R., et al., 'Revised definitions of women's sexual dysfunction' in *The Journal of Sexual Medicine*, 1 (July 2004), 40

Bell, S. E., 'Changing ideas: The medicalization of menopause' in *Social Science & Medicine* (1987), 24 (6) 535–42

Bullough, V., and Voght, M., 'Women, menstruation and nineteenth-century medicine' in *Bulletin of the History of Medicine*, 47 (1) (Spring 1973), 66–82

Cant, M. A., and Johnstone, R. A., 'Reproductive conflict and the separation of reproductive generations in humans' in *Proceedings of the National Academy of Science of the United States of America (PNAS)*, 31 March 2008

Cherry, K., Jamhour, N., and Mincey, P. B., review of Gullette, M., *Aged by Culture* in *Biography*, 27 (3) (Summer 2004), 631–4)

Chirawatkul, S., and Manderson, L., 'Perceptions of menopause in northeast Thailand: Contested meaning and practice' in *Social Science & Medicine* (1994), 39 (11), 1545–54

Crawford, P., 'Attitudes to Menstruation in seventeenth-century England' in *Past & Present*, 91 (May 1981), 47–73

Davis, S. R., Guay, A. T., Shifren, J. L., and Mazer, N. A., 'Endocrine aspects of female sexual dysfunction' in *The Journal of Sexual Medicine*, 1 (July 2004), 82

Dennerstein, L., and Hayes, R. D., 'The impact of aging on sexual function and sexual dysfunction in women: A review of population-based studies' in *The Journal of Sexual Medicine*, 2 (May 2005), 317

Dennerstein, L., and Hayes, R. D., 'Confronting the challenges: Epidemiological study of female sexual dysfunction and the menopause' in *The Journal of Sexual Medicine*, 2 (September 2005), 118

Dillaway, H. E., 'When does menopause occur, and how long does it last? Wrestling with age- and time-based conceptualizations of reproductive aging' in *NWSA* (National Women's Studies Association) *Journal*, 18 (1) (Spring 2006), 31–61

Featherstone, M., and Hepworth, M., 'The history of the male menopause 1848–1936' in *Maturitas* (1985), 7, 249–57

Feinson, M. C., 'Where are women in the history of aging?' in *Social Science History*, 9 (4) (Fall 1985), 429–52

Goldstein, I., and Alexander, J. L., 'Practical aspects in the management of vaginal atrophy and sexual dysfunction in perimenopausal and postmenopausal women' in *The Journal of Sexual Medicine*, 2 (September 2005), 154

Gould, D. C., Petty, R., and Jacobs, H. S., 'The male menopause – does it exist?' in *The British Medical Journal* (2000), 320, 858–61

Graziottin, A., and Leiblum, S. R., 'Biological and psychosocial pathophys-
iology of female sexual dysfunction during the menopausal
transition' in *The Journal of Sexual Medicine*, 2 (September 2005), 133

Groneman, C., 'Nymphomania: the historical construction of female sexuality' in *Signs: Journal of Women in Culture and Society*, 19 (2) (Winter 1994),
337–67.

Gurucharri, C. A., 'Culture and medical consultation' in *The Menopause at the
Millennium: Proceedings of the 9th International Menopause Society World Congress
on the Menopause* (London: Parthenon Publishing, 1999)

Heller, C. G., and Myers, G. B., 'The male climacteric, its symptomatology,
diagnosis and treatment' in *Journal of the American Medical Association*
(1944), 126, 472–7

Houck, J. A., '"What do these women want?": Feminist responses to *Feminine
Forever*, 1963–1980' in *Bulletin of the History of Medicine*, 77 (1) (Spring
2003), 103–32

Kent, S. K., 'Gender reconstruction after the First World War' in *British
Feminism in the Twentieth Century*, ed. Harold L. Smith (Aldershot: Edward
Elgar Publishing Ltd, 1990)

Lock, S., '"O that I were young again": Yeats and the Steinach Operation' in
British Medical Journal, 287 (24–31 December 1983), 1964–7

Lord, A., 'The great *Arcana* of the deity: Menstruation and menstrual disorders in eighteenth-century British medical thought' in *Bulletin of the
History of Medicine*, 73 (1) (Spring 1999), 38–63

MacPherson, K., 'Going to the source: Women reclaim menopause' in
Feminist Studies, 21 (2) (Summer 1995), 347

Magliano, D. J., Rogers, S. L., Abramson, M. J., and Tonkin, A. M., 'Hormone
therapy and cardiovascular disease: A systematic review and meta-
analysis' in *British Journal of Obstetrics and Gynaecology*, 113 (January 2006), 5

Micale, M. S., 'On the "disappearance" of hysteria: A study in the clinical
deconstruction of a diagnosis' in *Isis*, 84 (3) (September 1993), 496–526

Post, J. B., 'Ages at menarche and menopause: Some mediaeval authorities'
in *Population Studies* (1971), xxv, 83–7

Roberts, P. J., 'The menopause and hormone replacement therapy: Views of
women in general practice receiving hormone replacement therapy' in *British Journal of General Practice*, 41 (351) (October 1991), 421–4.

Scull, A., and Favreau, D., 'The cliterodectomy craze' in *Social Research*, 53 (2)
(Summer 1986), 243–60

Sengoopta, C., 'Secrets of eternal youth' in *History Today*, 56 (August 2006),
50–6

Shaw, S., 'Spontaneous combustion and the sectioning of female bodies' in *Literature and Medicine*, 14 (1) (Spring 1995), 1–22

Shorter, E., 'Women's diseases before 1900' in Albin, M. (ed.), with the assistance of Devlin, R. J., and Heeger, G., *New Directions in Psychohistory: The Adelphi Papers in Honor of Erik H. Erikson* (London: Allen Lane, 1983)

Smith-Rosenberg, C., 'Puberty to menopause: The cycle of femininity in nineteenth-century America' in *Feminist Studies*, 1 (3–4) (Winter–Spring 1973), 58–72

Stolberg, M., 'A woman's hell? Medical perceptions of menopause in pre-industrial Europe' in *Bulletin of the History of Medicine* (1999), 73, 404–28

Strange, J-M., 'Menstrual fictions: Languages of medicine and menstruation, c. 1850–1930' in *Women's History Review* (2000), 9 (3), 607–28.

Theriot, N. M., 'Women's voices in nineteenth-century medical discourse: A step toward deconstructing science' in *Signs*, 19 (1) (Autumn 1993), 1–31

Wear, A., 'Making sense of health and the environment in early modern England' in Wear, A. (ed.), *Medicine in Society* (Cambridge: CUP, 1992)

Wilbush, J., 'Tilt, E. J. and the change of life (1857) – the only work on the subject in the English language' in *Maturitas* (1980), 2, 259–67

Winterich, J. A., 'Sex, menopause, and culture: Sexual orientation and the meaning of menopause for women's sex lives' in *Gender & Society*, 17 (4) (August 2003), 627–42

Websites

International Menopause Society – http://www.imsociety.org

Oxford Reference Online – http://www.oxfordreference.com/views/ENTRY.html?subview=Main&entry=t38.e1810

INDEX